Plague Houses and Pandemics.

Alison Wall

Published by New Generation Publishing in 2023

Copyright © Alison Wall 2023

First Edition

The author asserts the moral right under the Copyright, Designs and Patents Act 1988 to be identified as the author of this work.

All Rights reserved. No part of this publication may be reproduced, stored in a retrieval system or transmitted, in any form or by any means without the prior consent of the author, nor be otherwise circulated in any form of binding or cover other than that which it is published and without a similar condition being imposed on the subsequent purchaser.

ISBN: 978-1-83563-023-5

www.newgeneration-publishing.com

New Generation Publishing

For Felix

Acknowledgements

I would like to thank the following for their generous help and support writing this book.

Lucy Dalton for her enthusiasm about the subject and help with information about a local Pest House, Mike Kemp for signposting me to relevant books and other sources and Annie Unwin for making contact with the owners of Hitchin Pest House. Jonathan and Emily Read for generously sharing information about their home and its history. I would like to thank Isabel Thompson at Hertfordshire County Council for sending through a detailed list of Hertfordshire Pest Houses.

In particular I would like to acknowledge and thank Patricia Maunder for proofreading the work and for her eye for detail.

For Tony, who has encouraged me to keep going, helped with technical difficulties and supported me throughout. The work on this book came to a halt last year, but thanks to a dear friend Alison Allard it got back on track and has at last been completed.

I would also like to thank my dear daughter-in-law Rachael and son Jon, for helping me to persevere with the images in this book.

Every attempt has been made to seek permission for copyright material used in this book. However, the author wishes to apologise if I have inadvertently used copyright material without permission and acknowledgement. I will make the necessary correction at the first opportunity.

I dedicate this book to Felix, Archie and Alex and all of their generation in the hope that as they grow up they will treasure our historic buildings and the stories they have to tell. Sadly so many historic building have been demolished, with areas losing their character and charm. I hope in particular that those Pest Houses still standing will be lovingly cared for, for future generations.

Alison Wall. 2023

Contents

Acknowledgements	iv
Plague Houses and Pandemics.	1
1 - Introduction	3
2 - The Black Death 1348	11
3 - Beliefs about the cause of plague	13
4 - 'Cures' for the plague – medical, herbal and religious	21
5 - Quarantine	38
6 - Pavage and sanitation – the changing urban environment.	41
7 - Events leading up to 1665	44
8 - The Story of Eyam	59
9 - The pest house system	69
10 - Pest Houses demolished in England.	82
11 - Pest Houses still standing.	95
12 - Isolation hospitals and fever nursing.	107
13 - Similarities and Differences in health protection between 1665 and 2020	126
14 - Reflections	132
APPENDIX 1 Shakespeare's plays that allude to the plague.	136
APPENDIX 2: The Diary of Samuel Pepys. Edited by R.C.Latham & W.Matthews. Vol.V1. 1665	141
APPENDIX 3: History and development of the Hitchin Pest House.	143
END NOTES	150

Plague Houses and Pandemics.

Thomas Nashe (1592)
A Litany in Time of Plague
ADIEU, farewell, earth's bliss;
This world uncertain is;
Fond are life's lustful joys;
Death proves them all but toys;
I am sick, I must die.

Lord, have mercy on us!
Rich men, trust not wealth,
Gold cannot buy you health;
Physic himself must fade.
All things to end are made,
The plague full swift goes by;
I am sick I must die

Lord have mercy on us!
Beauty is but a flower
Which wrinkels will devour;
Brightness falls from the air;
Queens have died young and fair;
Dust hath closed Helen's eye.
I am sick, I must die.

Lord, have mercy on us.
Strength stoops unto the grave,
Worms feed on Hector brave;
Swords may not fight with fate,

Earth still holds ope her gate.
"Come, come!" the bells do cry.
I am sick, I must die.

Lord, have mercy on us.
   Haste, therefore, each degree,
   To welcome destiny;
   Heaven is our heritage,
   Earth but a player's stage;
   Mount we unto the sky.
   I am sick, I must die.

Lord, have mercy on us.

Chapter One - Introduction

Why write about pestilence/ plague (pest) houses, and what are they? What was so special about the reign of Charles II and what did our Merrie Monarch actually do?

I will refer to these houses as either pest, pestilence or plague cottages throughout the book. The term pest is derived from the French 'La Peste' which translates to the plague. [1]

Seventeen years ago I was working as a museum guide when a colleague raised the subject of Pest Houses. He was convinced that Pest Houses were for diseased cattle. I felt sure that somewhere I had read about them as places to remove those suffering from plague and small pox. It's true that cattle plague was a widespread problem [2] but there is no evidence that cattle were managed in this way. I started to search for information and became fascinated with the role of Pest Houses in the evolution of public health history. Pest Houses have been used since Tudor times to accommodate those with plague and smallpox. I could not find one book that described these places in detail, except references to them in general texts. In this book, I discuss the evolution of public health from the Pest Houses to modern day management of pandemics.

I include the details I have obtained from various sources and describe the Pestilence Houses I have been able to visit. I have struggled to find any clear material that discusses the outcomes of care and segregation in Pest Houses, but it seems that some sufferers did survive as a result of being attended to in a warm and dry environment.

Pest Houses will be described within the context of the changing patterns of belief about health and disease. The text will explain how a coordinated approach was achieved within communities after the Edict issued by Charles II in 1665.

I will argue that in the time of the reign of Charles II, he had the foresight to adopt a public health perspective, which has become embedded today in sophisticated public health policy making.

I challenge you to consider when public health as a concept was adopted in Britain and what we mean exactly by the term public health? This book discusses the evolution of public health from the medieval to the modern.

Specific Pestilence (Pest) Houses will be described, both those that are no longer standing and those that remain. Their functions will be detailed, looking in particular at the role they served in isolating the plague and caring for those with smallpox. The main focus will centre on London, where the scale of infections was the greatest.

There appears to be considerable confusion about the designation of Pest Houses, as they have been labelled as the village's poor house or workhouse, with no knowledge that they served a public health purpose in society centuries ago. Monastic records were mostly destroyed during the Reformation under Henry VIII. The Great Fire of London in 1666 resulted in some parish records being lost, including the records kept in the library of the College of Physicians in Warwick Lane. Why has so little been written about the Pest Houses? It may well be that people wanted to forget the terrible experiences they endured. We are indebted to contemporaries such as Henry Foe, John Allin and Samuel Pepys (1633 – 1703), who had the foresight to record details of the seventeenth century plague years. Henry Foe wrote about the system for containment of the plague, which was surprisingly well developed for that time. An apothecary William Boghurst and a doctor, Nathaniel Hodges, also had the foresight to write about the clinical details of their work, which I shall discuss later.

I move on to the creation of fever hospitals and the training of fever nurses, as a response to the rising problem of infectious diseases, such as diphtheria and scarlet fever.

Pandemics then and now will be compared, with a view towards future infection containment. We can learn so much from the practice of removing people to Pest Houses, since the

Elizabethan era. We can also learn a lot about human behaviour and understand better why people react as they do to regulation and restraint. The role of the State versus individual freedom is another dilemma to face amidst a complexity of moral choices. It is inevitable that we will face future pandemics with the rise of more virulent infections. In the past we have witnessed at least fifty million dying worldwide form the Spanish flu in 1918 and more recently we have had Severe Acute Respiratory Syndrome (SARS), with the horseshoe bat being the natural reservoir for the virus. It is recorded that it infected more than 8000 people and killed 774. It was traced to the palm civet. Middle East Respiratory Syndrome (MERS) was traced to infected camels, again likely to have caught the virus from bats. About 2500 people have caught the virus, with a thirty-five per cent mortality rate. Covid 19 has killed millions and is thought also to have originated in horseshoe bats. We need to learn from history and prepare as best we can for what lies ahead. I believe that we need the isolation hospitals again, so we can segregate the infectious from chronic conditions and cancers.

I hope you will become as fascinated with these houses as I have and that those houses that remain will be listed for the future as valued heritage assets. Too many have been lost and those that remain need the recognition they deserve.

I aim to convince you that the public health movement did not originate in the nineteenth century, as most people believe, with the laying down of sewers and industrialisation on a grand scale. The principles of public health were espoused centuries ago at the time of Henry VIII, but it was during the reign of Charles II when he published his Edict concerning the Great Plague, to ensure a co-ordinated and standardised approach to disease containment that a co-ordinated system was set in place.

This is the story of the evolution of public health care, starting with the little known primitive Pest House, to the sophisticated state of the art institutions, like the Nightingale Hospitals.

What do we mean by the term public health?

Public Health is defined as "the art and science of preventing disease, prolonging life and promoting health through the organized efforts of society" [3]. There are a number of other definitions, but the basis of public health is adopting a community focus.

Communities need to define their priority issues, and adopt a strategic view.

An entity such as a community health management system needs to select the priorities, make decisions and create a community-wide population health learning system. In other words a structure is required to be set in place.

The culture, values and beliefs about health and disease of the time will determine how public health practices are established. Technology will drive the mechanisms of achieving the public health goals laid out.

Public health is all to do with improving the health and wellbeing of communities. It is not simply the provision of medical services, but involves the availability of appropriate facilities and resources. People need to feel well as well as be physically well. Communities require green and open spaces and community facilities, so that they feel part of a wider societal network. John Evelyn wrote about the importance of green spaces and can be seen as the first environmentalist in Britain. [4] (*Fumifugium/Silva* 1661). His ideas paved the way for the much later creation of garden cities designed by Ebenezer Howard. Individuals seek a sense that they have a role to play and purpose in their community. One of the aims of public health is to understand where the inequalities in health lie and put in resources to promote a narrowing between varying health experiences. So in essence public health is a multi-disciplinary approach. The local authority plays a significant part, alongside such services as dentistry, ophthalmology, secondary health care and companies such as water companies, who control the quality of our water supplies.

What have been some key public health achievements over time?

Many infectious diseases are now controlled

through rigorous vaccination programmes, or have been eradicated altogether like smallpox. Edward Jenner discovered the smallpox vaccine with others, through his research into cow pox in 1796. Details of his achievements will be described in a later chapter.

Sir Alexander Fleming discovered penicillin in 1928. Some also ascribe the discovery to a Frenchman Ernest Duchesne, who made notes about the antibiotic qualities of 'penicillin glaucun' in 1897. [5] The Scottish physician at St. Mary's, Paddington and Nobel Laureate returned from his holiday to find his petri dishes of staphylococcus bacteria contaminated with mould. The mould (penicillin) had destroyed the bacteria. The first person in the world to receive penicillin was a British policeman on 12 February 1941. Two years later Fleming was knighted for his discovery.

Heart disease and stroke risks are understood to be linked to lifestyle choices, and risks reduce with smoking cessation, exercise and healthier eating. Stress plays an important part in health outcomes, with stress causing such conditions as high blood pressure and digestive disorders.

We now enjoy safer and healthier foods due to more refined food processing, refrigeration and preservation methods. Fluoridisation of drinking water is directly related to improved dental health and reduced caries.

Road and home safety initiatives have resulted in fewer accidents, with the introduction for example of speed restrictions, smoke and carbon monoxide monitors.

These are all examples of how public health and wellbeing has resulted in better health outcomes for communities.

Chapter Two - The Black Death 1348

The Black Death arrived in Europe in 1347. Trading ships pulled into the port of Messina in Sicily, with clear signs that many of the sailors were dying of the plague. They were coughing up blood and had oozing boils on their bodies. [1]

The account of the first infection comes from the writings of a Franciscan friar Michael of Piazza. [2] The sickness spread across Europe, with indiscriminate effects. Young and old, rich and poor died in their millions. The belief was that it was the wrath of God taking vengeance for their sins.

As with the coronavirus pandemic, it was thought it originated in Asia. There were accounts of outbreaks in various European countries prior to 1347. However, the plague could spread quickly along trading routes, particularly the Silk Road and by sea.

The plague *'found awaiting it in Europe a population singularly ill-equipped to resist.'* [3]

The plague arrived in England the following year by sea, via the trade routes. [4] Giovanni Boccaccio, an Italian writer described the buboes or tumours as being as large as eggs. They appeared where the lymph nodes are under the armpits, neck and groin. Other symptoms were vomiting, coughing up blood and fever. The worst year in England was 1349, with the writings on the walls of St. Mary's Church, Ashwell in Hertfordshire testifying to the

'Wretched, terrible, destructive year, the remnants of the people alone remain.'

Nothing is known about the victims, although it's estimated a third to a half of the population died. They were thrown indiscriminately into a local pit in Mill Street, Ashwell [5]

Waves of plague brought terror to communities, but medieval society was more inured to human disasters than is the case today. They learnt to live with it.

The whole country never again was as overwhelmed with infection as it was in the period of 1348-9. Afterwards there were outbreaks in different parts of the country. The plague of 1361 *(pestis pueronum)* principally affected the young and the upper classes. It is thought possibly this occurred as the young had mostly escaped the plague twelve years earlier.

Quarantine lazzarettos, named after St. Lazarus, were deployed to safeguard trade routes. Old leper hospitals were requisitioned and the first Pest House was built at Ragusa,Dubrovnik in 1377, while Venice enforced quarantine on the lagoon Islands in 1423 [6] Venice was a key trading route and economic hub, therefore protection against disease was critical [7].

Chapter Three - Beliefs about the cause of plague

What exactly was the plague or pestilence?

In the early seventeenth century the general belief was that there were organisms or seeds in the air that caused plague. [1] Leeuwenhoek discovered the *infusoria, or tiny micrto-orgsanisdms in water* [2]. He believed little animals in the air were the causative organisms [3].

Thomas Sherwood, a Practitioner in Physick in 1641 believed that there were

'divers caufes of this difeafe.' [4].

In order of priority he listed

'the firft is fin, the fecund an infected and corrupted air, the third an evill diet and the fourth are evill humours.' (The f's are s's in post medieval English).

He stated that these causes were applicable to both the plague and smallpox. He listed his suggested remedies, addressing each in turn and included the practice of bloodletting, repentance of all sins, changes in diet and the use of chemicals.

It has been suggested that the infection could have been influenza, smallpox, typhus or even anthrax. However we now know that the plague is caused by a bacterium called *Yersinia pestis.* It was discovered by Yersin in Hong Kong in 1894. It is a gram negative coccobacillus. It is transmitted via infected fleas. The accepted view has been that rats transmitted the infection and passed it on to blood sucking fleas, but other rodents like gerbils may have been responsible as well. Fleas and body lice can lodge themselves in cloth, grain and clothing and this is how the village of Eyam got infected, which I describe in a later chapter.

Several years after Yersin's discovery researchers in India identified the rat as the vector, with a zoonotic jump from flea to rat to human. It is spread by the bite of a rat's flea, which is a parasite of the black rat, *rattus rattus*. The flea feeds on the blood of its infected host and the ingested bacilli multiply blocking the proventriculus, the organ at the entrance to the flea's stomach. If the flea bites and attempts to feed on a human, the passage of blood into the flea's stomach is obstructed by the blocked proventriculus and so is regurgitated, carrying the plague bacillus into its human host. The rat's flea requires relatively high temperatures and humidity; essentially, the greater the humidity the lower the temperature in which it can survive. The ideal conditions seem to be ninety to ninety-five per cent humidity and temperatures of around 15 to 25 degrees centigrade. The microclimates provided by a rat's nest, or woollen-cloth, or stocks of grain, probably would have provided the necessary conditions. The black rat lived close to human habitations and is a climber, and so could get to upper floors and into roofs, and feed on grain. Control or exterminate the rat and you can limit the spread of bubonic plague. [5]. Strangely, the fleas are very attracted to white objects, but can be repelled by certain strong smells [6]. After the death of the host the flea has three days to find a new source of blood.

The picture is more complicated than simple transmission from rat to human. Though many fleas can become infected, it is only a minority that go on to become infective. [7]

It may be that the plague can be transmitted without the intervention of the rat as a vector [8], as the spread of disease can be so rapid through close human bodily contact. More recent research [9] has discovered that the plague in Glasgow and other cities like Liverpool in 1900 was spread from human to human through infected body lice (*pediculus humanus humanus*) and the human flea (*pulex irritans*). There is no evidence that it was from rat transmission. [10]. The slums and tenements of Glasgow and Liverpool were not that different from the slums of London in 1665. One would expect that if the plague was transmitted solely by rats that the outbreak would have started near the ports and docks, when in fact the initial outbreak of the Great Plague in London was in Drury Lane, in the parish of St. Giles in the Fields.

The plague presents itself in three distinct forms, named after their most obvious characteristic:

bubonic (buboes or swellings are present), pneumonic (a virulent form which occurs when the infection moves into the lungs) and septicaemic (the bacteria enters and infects the bloodstream). The bubonic plague has an incubation period of one to six days. The bubonic plague destroys the lymphatic system, the body's line of defence. [11] This results in fever, seizures and extreme muscle pain. Huge walnut sized buboes would erupt in the lymph nodes, the neck and groin being the commonest sites. Gangrene would spread and the nose would blacken through lack of circulating blood. Once the disease reached the lungs of the malnourished, it then spread to the wider population through sneezes and coughs. The mortality rate of the bubonic plague varied between forty to eighty per cent [12]. Pneumonic plague led to about ninety per cent mortality, and in the rarer septiceamic plague the death rate was hundred per cent. Most victims died three to ten days after initial infection, although in the case of pneumonic and septiceamic plague victims died quickly, within one or two days. A mild form of the plague has been documented [13]. This is termed *pestis minor.* By the seventeenth century pneumonic plague seems to have been in abeyance, with the bubonic form in high prevalence.

Fleas were commonplace and particularly the poor learnt to live with them. John Donne (1572-1631) wrote a poem called the Flea-

*'It sucked me first and now sucks thee
And in this flea our two bloods mingled be'*
[14]

The people believed that disease befell them because of their sinfulness. The physician William Bullein was the first English man of the sixteenth century to fuse the spiritual and corporal [15]. It was believed that sinfulness could be breathed in and out, carried by insects shot through the air by elf shot. Satan was also known as Beelzebub or "Lord of the Flies".

Daniel Defoe (1661 -1731) in 1722, wrote up the notes left by his uncle Henry Foe, in *'A Journal of a Plague Year'*. Henry worked as a butcher in the East End of London. He made the decision not to move away from London, despite protestations from his brother and he provides graphic detail of life and death in the City during 1665 [16]

Defoe explains that [17]

'we draw in breath when we breath, and therefore 'tis the hand of God; there is no withstanding it.'

Some turned to flagellation. Flagellants whipped and beat themselves as an act of penance to God.

'Except for occasional hymns, the marchers were silent, with their heads bowed.' [18].

However the practice was not common in England, or approved by the Church. Fasting was also practised, seeking God's forgiveness through self-discipline and restraint.

The great philosophers and physicians Hippocrates (c460 – 357BC) Claudius Galen (c129-199AD) and Aristotle (384-322 BC) were the founding fathers of early thoughts on disease. Aristotle was the first to use the theory of four humours, which was further developed by Hippocrates. The writings of Hippocrates were actually written by a collective and influenced medical practice for over 2000 years [19] Hippocrates beliefs were based on three principles. Sickness could be explained scientifically and was not divine intervention, there is a need to balance humours to restore health and thirdly nature is its own best healer. Galen developed the early Hippocratic teachings and used pulse readings as a basis for diagnosis.

The humours were thought to be a matrix linking fluid elements throughout the body, thereby determining personality types. We still talk about being in good and bad humour.

Yellow bile in excess resulted they believed in a choleric personality (hot and dry) fiery personality associated with the summer months.

An imbalance of phlegm caused someone to be cold and moist. This humoral type is linked to water and cold winters

Black bile imbalance resulted in a melancholic character (cold and dry) related to the earth and the autumn.

Too much blood was linked to a sanguine type of person, being hot and moist (air). The season of spring is linked to blood and excess blood was believed to be a symptom of the plague. Bloodletting was seen as restorative to reduce heat and fever.

Star signs were mapped to parts of the body, for example it was thought that Scorpio controlled the reproductive organs. Melancholy was associated with Saturn, because the planet was believed to be slow moving [20]

Shakespeare describes the four personality types in his plays. (See Appendix 1) All four personality types appear in *'Henry IV'*. A person who was hot tempered and easily angered was said to be choleric and two choleric characters are the lead players in *'Taming of the Shrew'*. Peruchio attempts to control Kate by starving her and cooling her humours.

By the 1620's William Harvey, a member of the Royal Society, had discovered the elementary circulation of the blood. As with all new theories it took some time for the established beliefs to be discarded and new theories accepted.

Dekker believed that people's emotional state was related to whether they succumbed to the plague or not. He proposed that laughter was the best antidote and that those who were

'melancholy for the loss of friends were predisposed to it, whilst cheerfulness and courage fortified some against it' [21].

Defoe in *'A Journal of a Plague Year'* talks about common beliefs. He states *'talk about the infection being carried on by the air only, by carrying with it vast numbers of insects and invisible creatures, who enter into the body with the breath, or even the pores, and there generate most acute poisons, or poisonous ovae.'* [22]

As it was believed that the plague passed through the skin via open skin pores, so sweating was seen as the best initial remedy as Daniel Defoe describes

'the ordinary remedy to be taken when the first apprehension of the distemper began'

Over time it began to be recognised that the plague could lie dormant in the soil and then erupt when conditions permitted in warmer weather. But in 1665 the plague dead were buried in shallow graves, as there was no awareness of this risk. A combination of overcrowding, soil contamination and warm weather all contributed to regular outbreaks over the centuries.

Today plague continues to strike communities. Modern outbreaks are still concentrated in Africa and parts of Asia. [23/24]

Chapter Four - 'Cures' for the plague – medical, herbal and religious

The generally accepted tenet was that the pestilence was carried in the air – the miasmic theory of disease. It could be local, for example a swamp, or cover a wide area. It could also be temporary, as a result of some disturbance. In fact the miasmic theory was not discounted until the Victorian period, when the germ theory of disease, postulated by Robert Koch, was eventually accepted. At the time of Florence Nightingales' death in 1910 both the miasmic theory and germ theory formed the basis of medical practice.

In 1665 Charles II turned to the Royal College of Physicians for advice. The Royal College at this time was well respected, having been established in 1518 to cover the City of London, in the reign of Henry VIII. The College was granted a Royal Charter in 1523, by which time the College regulated physicians across the whole of England. . A small group of physicians, headed up by Thomas Linacre, persuaded the King in 1518 that a College should be founded, to standardise medical care and to provide some degree of regulation of practice.

There were basically two schools of thought, namely the Galenists and the Paracelsists, after the ancient alchemist Paracelsus (1493 -1541). Paracelsists believed that disease arose from dysfunctional chemical processes. They believed three active substances determined health and balance, namely mercury, sulphur and salt. [1]. The Galenists followed the teachings of Galen, the second century Greek physician. He believed in herbal and natural remedies. The Galenists were scorned by the Paracelists for their practices of bleeding, purging and vomiting. Sometimes theories were combined, resulting in pluralism of thought.

Sir.Theodore Mayerne, (1573-1655) physician to James I and Charles I, was one of the first to adopt the chemical approach, so following the school of Paracelsus. He advised the use of such concoctions as calomel and blackwash. Calomel was a mix of mercury and chlorine. When mixed with limewater, it was known as blackwash.

To protect themselves from stinking air the followers of Galen carried sweet smelling nosegays and herbs. Civet boxes, containing liquid from civet cats produced sweet smelling perfume and pouncet boxes had pierced holes through which the smells from a sponge soaked in vinegar could emanate. The medieval physic garden was deemed to be an important source of sweet smelling remedies for various ills, including the plague. A notable herbalist John

Gerard (1545 – 1612), a member of the Barber-Surgeons, became the curator of the physic garden of the College of Physicians in 1586 and held his position until 1604. He wrote *The Herball or general Historie of Plantes* in 1597, detailing the medicinal uses of herbs found across the world. [2] Another contemporary was Sir Thomas Browne (1605-1682) doctor and naturalist who studied the properties of plants. He communicated regularly with John Evelyn. His most famous work is *Pseudo Doxia Epidemica* [3] Browne distinguished religion from science and believed in a holistic view of health and wellbeing, including the biosocial and spiritual.

Helen Steadman in her book *'Widdershins'* explains that medieval belief centred on the theory that like cures like. Bare elderberry sprigs for example resembled the branches of the lung, so it was believed that elder was the best cure for respiratory complaints. [4] This is now known as "*The Theory of Signatures.*"

Following the humoral and paracelsists, bloodletting became a favoured practice. Drawing blood was used to restore balance to the four humours. Leeches were used as a gentler method, or the more painful method of cutting the skin and veins to remove several pints of blood. The bush broom was treated to make beer, to induce a degree of sweating. It was believed that sweating opened up the skin pores to allow the escape of the plague particles.

Another cure sometimes reserved for the wealthy was to crush emeralds down to a fine powder and mix into food. Trying to swallow it however would be the same as trying to bite into glass.

Other practices involved bathing in urine, rubbing tree resin into the skin, flower roots and faeces were liberally applied directly onto the oozing sores. The pungent smell of onions was believed to purify the air and toads were placed on suppurating buboes [5]

A vast array of potions were concocted and prescribed.

Defoe's observations from the time really illustrate this –

'almost every physician prescribes or prepares a different thing, as his judgement or experience guides him.' [6].

Defoe mentions a mixture called *Venice treacle*. It was acclaimed as the anti-pestilential pill [6] or cure all. [7]

In fact the main internal remedies for the plague were London treacle, mithridatium, galene and diascordium. Diascordium was a confection prepared from the water germander. Water germander (*Tencrium Scordium*) grows in marshy areas in Europe and today is a rare species in Britain. Rubbing the leaves together releases a penetrating odour similar to garlic. Little is known of its side effects or how it works. On occasions it was made with opium. Surgeons or chirigeons were known to lance buboes and then wash them with such potions as London treacle.

Mithridatium and diascordium were listed in the authoritative formulary of the time '*Pharmacopoeia Londinensis'* printed in 1618.

Nicholas Culpeper (1616-1654) a Galenist and famous herbalist in 1649 wrote in his dispensatory about mithridatium and Venetian treacle and advocated their use. He believed that seven 'naturals' were required to be healthy, namely humours, spirits, elements, complexions, members, virtues and operations. [8]. Culpeper also believed that herbs were governed by planetary motions, for example the mulberry tree was ruled by Mercury. This meant that he believed herbal effects were variable according to where the planets were in the solar system. Culpeper felt it was important that the ordinary person could understand the workings of the vast array of medicinal herbs and not be subject to paying high fees to the physicians. In 1649 he translated the Royal College of Physicians tome called the *Pharmacopoeia Londinesis* into plain English, published as *A Physical Directory.* This predictably totally enraged the College of Physicians. [9]

Mithridatium is named after Mithridates VI of Pontus in 120 BC. He was the first known experimental toxicologist and concocted the mixture. *Mithridatium* was heralded as a universal panacea for centuries, until it came into disrepute after the concerns raised by William Heberden in

1745. He was concerned about their likely toxicity. Eventually modern medical regulation resulted in the discontinuation of use of these remedies, as more understanding of their potency was discovered.

Galene is named after the philosopher and physician Galen. Galen adapted mixtures with vipers flesh in the second century AD, when he was physician to the Roman Emperor Marcus Aurelius. The name *galene* translated means tranquillity. It was a complex mixture, comprising over fifty five ingredients.

Both *mithridatium* and *galene* were recommended to be taken orally, with either water or wine. They were also used topically on the skin or even used on the eye.

Hermione Eyre has written a fascinating account of the seventeenth century muse Venetia Stanley and her alchemist husband, Sir Kenelm Digby [10]. In 1633 Venetia was discovered dead in bed. No one could agree why she had died, but she had consumed a beauty tonic called 'Viper Wine' or *Benzoardicum Thericale*. This originated in Venice and her husband Digby had a recipe for it. It seems likely that she developed a dependency on it. Hers was a short life, dying at the age of only thirty two years. This in depth investigation into her death illustrates how alchemists mixed a range of unproven herbs and chemicals and laid great store on the merits of vipers flesh.

As it was believed that plague was carried in

the air, notably the south wind, some resorted to hiding in caves and sewers to avoid the stench of the air.

Other beliefs involved the drinking of arsenic and mercury, sitting next to sulphurous fires, or attaching live farm animals and toads to a victim in the hope that the infection would pass from man to animal.

Defoe describes how the Lord Mayor ordered the College of Physicians to

'publish directions for cheap remedies for the poor' [11]. It seems therefore that the more exotic preparations described were reserved for the aristocracy and upper classes, who could afford to pay for these potions.

In 1665 Dr Francis Glisson (1597-1677) recommended as his 'constant antidote' a piece of dried manure of someone who had died of the disease, kept in a house in a porous box for 'the best antidote perfume'. Many of the nostrums and antidotes were unconvincing, and this one in particular sounds like the advice of a crank or at least an eccentric, but Glisson was a Cambridge man, who was Regius Professor of Physic for more than 40 years, a Fellow of the College of Physicians and an original fellow of the Royal Society. [12]

Vinegar was commonly used by the poor, as it was easily available and a cheap commodity. Again Defoe says one poor lady

'washed her head in vinegar and sprinkled

her head clothes so with vinegar ....she sniffed vinegar up her nose and held a handkerchief wetted with vinegar to her mouth.' [13].

Vinegar was used as the general disinfectant and evidence for disinfecting coins can be seen when visiting the plague village of Eyam in Derbyshire. The image shows the boundary stone between the villages of Eyam and Stoney Middleton, where villagers left their money in exchange for essential provisions.

The practice of burning fires was controversial; physicians advised this as a way to rid homes of the plague, even in the summer months. This is consistent with the belief that sweating helped to open skin pores for the disease to dissipate. As we will see in a later chapter most of the Pest Houses at the time had prominent chimneys. However others were sceptical of this, as they believed that heating the blood would increase the distemper, as the plague numbers rose during the warm summer months. Burning fires was at odds with the beliefs of John Evelyn, a fellow of the Royal Society who believed that fires should be restricted to areas outside the City and he compared the health of London to that of Paris, where industry was not permitted in the city. Public and private fires were burnt as Pepys details in his daily diary recordings. Also Defoe writes that there was

'one at Custom House,, one at Billingsgate,

one at Queenhith, and one at the Three Cranes, one in Blackfriars, and one at the gate of Brideswell'.[14]

Pepys also believed that head shaving would help and periwigs became fashionable, as long as the wig hair came from a safe source.

Surgeons also used heat on the swellings or buboes to encourage them to rupture. Foul smelling black serum would then drain away and some survived after this practice. Defoe describes this as

'The terrible burnings of the caustics' [15]

Tobacco, smoked or chewed, came into great vogue in 1665 as a preventative from the plague. In fact it was the most popular remedy. Hearne, the antiquary, says:

'I have been told that in the last great plague at London [1665] none that kept tobacconists shops had the plague. It is certain that smoaking it was looked upon as a most excellent preservative; in so much that even children were obliged to smoak. And I remember that I heard formerly Tom Rogers, who was yeoman beadle, say that when he was that year, when the plague raged, a schoolboy at Eaton, all the boys of that school were obliged to smoak in the school every morning, and that he was never whipped so much in his life as he was one morning for not smoaking.' [16]

Pepys also took to chewing tobacco as a preventative [17]

Adherents to the humoral theory advocated a sense of cheerfulness to combat the plague. Both William Boghurst (1630 – 1685) and Nathaniel Hodges (1629-1688) recommended a lifestyle of company, a pint of sack daily and musick. This would counterbalance the melancholic humour.

People would also resort to magic and witchcraft and cast spells in the hope of salvation. The chanting of ABRACADABRA would be heard in the streets. Pedlars increased their sale of charms, philtres (magic potions), exorcisms, signs of the zodiac and amulets. Others believed there was cabalistic significance to the year 1666. They made reference to the words in Revelation –

'the number of the beast …his number is six hundred, three score and six.' [18]

At the time of the Great Plague of 1665, England was on the cusp between the following of magic and scientific theories. There was a convergence of both the magical and the scientific in the way that people tried to control and treat the contagion.

From the writings and beliefs of Galen, Aristotle and Hippocrates there arose the empirical method, which involved learning through experience and experiment.

Limewash was used to clean the houses of those afflicted and then the building was fumigated using a mix of brimstone, saltpetre and sulphur. Mixing these produces sulphur dioxide. Experiments have been conducted to test their efficacy and remarkably using lime wash and fumigation killed fleas and body lice [19]. Scientists have discovered that the body louse can transmit both plague and typhus. They can crawl up to five metres in one day. Carbon dioxide in our exhaled breath wakes them up to feed and reproduce, so their activity is a real challenge to address.

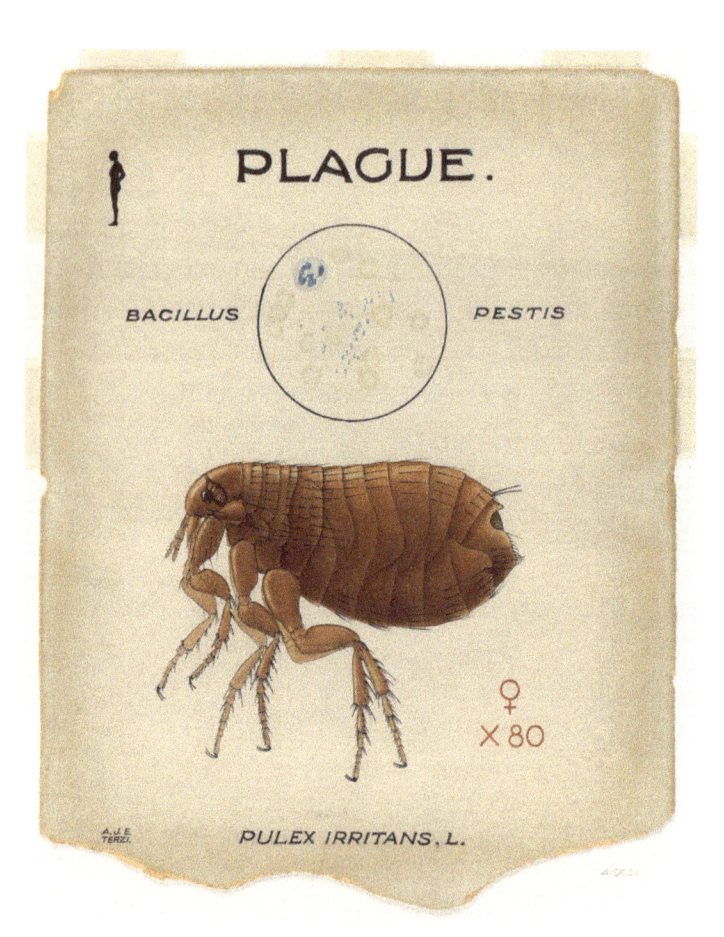

Bacillus pestis
Wellcome Collection

Bill of Mortality
Wellcome Collection

FUMIFUGIUM:

OR

The Inconveniencie of the AER
AND
SMOAK of LONDON
DISSIPATED.

TOGETHER

With some REMEDIES humbly
PROPOSED

By J. E. Esq;

To His Sacred MAJESTIE,
AND
To the PARLIAMENT now Assembled.

Published by His Majesties Command.

Lucret. l. 5.
Carbonúmque gravis vis, atque odor insinuatur
Quam facile in cerebrum?

LONDON,
Printed by W. Godbid for Gabriel Bedel, and Thomas Collins,
and are to be sold at their Shop at the Middle Temple Gate
neer Temple-Bar. M. DC. LXI.

Fumifugium and smoak of London
Wellcome Collection

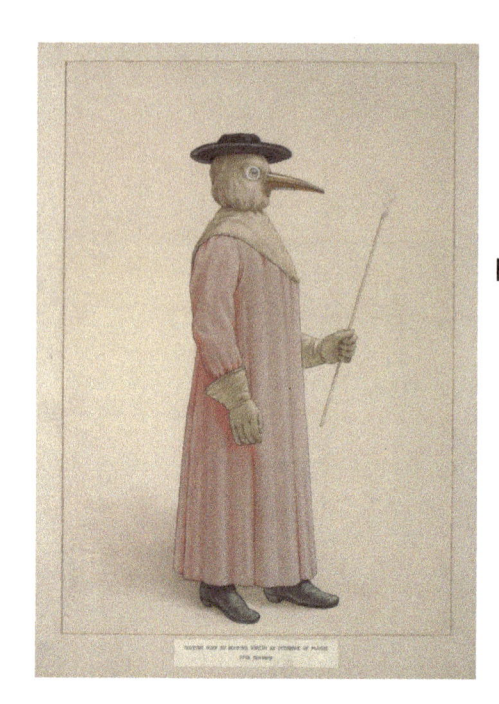

Plague Doctor
Look and Learn

Plague Street
Look and Learn

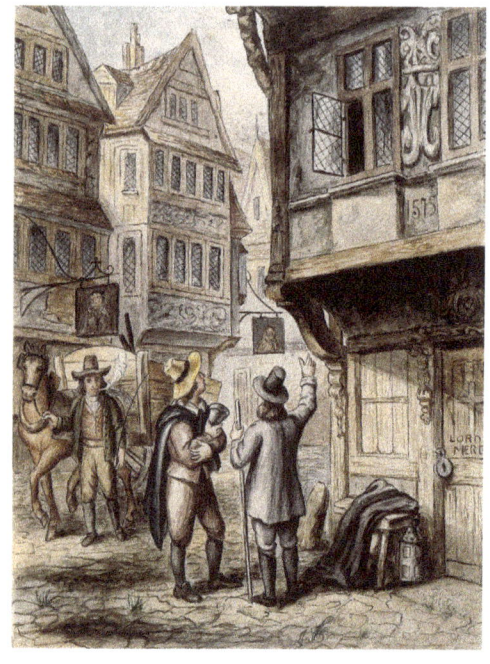

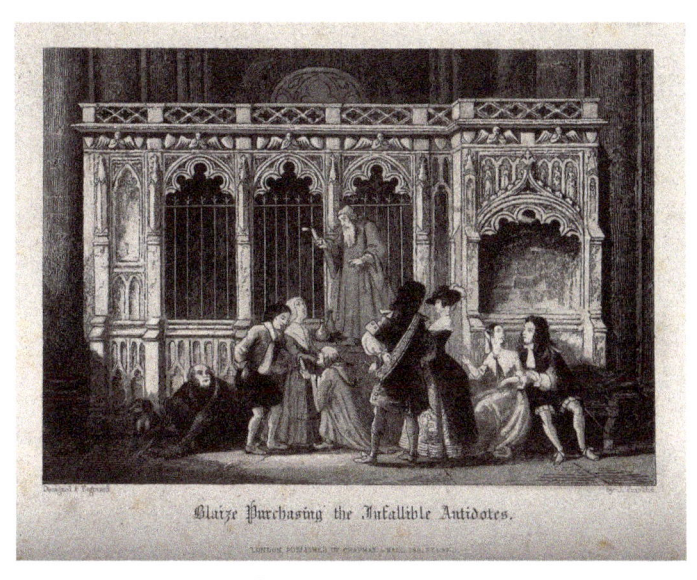

Infallible antidotes
Look and Learn

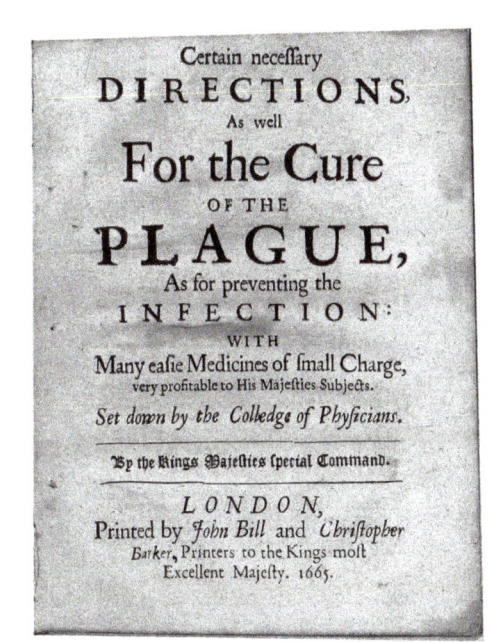

Directions for the cure of the plague
Look and Learn

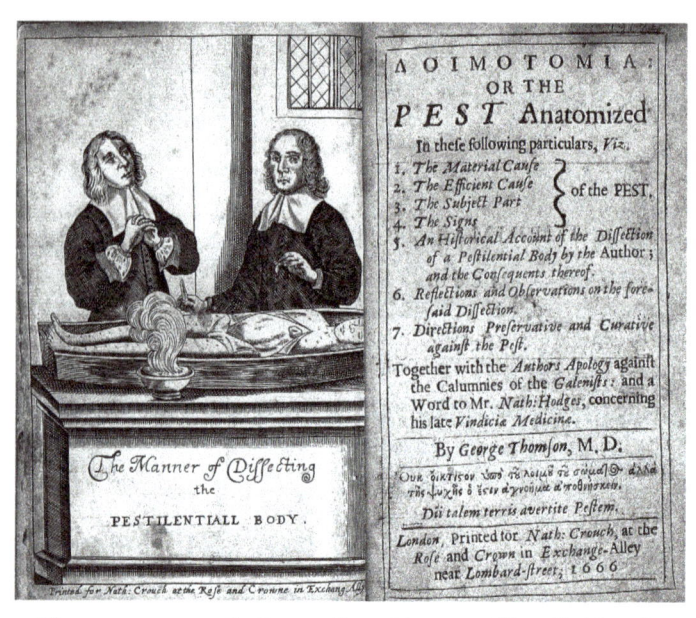

The manner of dissecting the pestilential body
Look and Learn

Amulets and quackery
Look and Learn

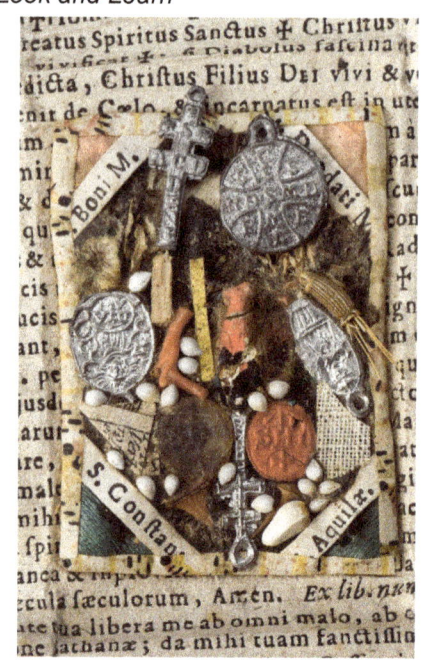

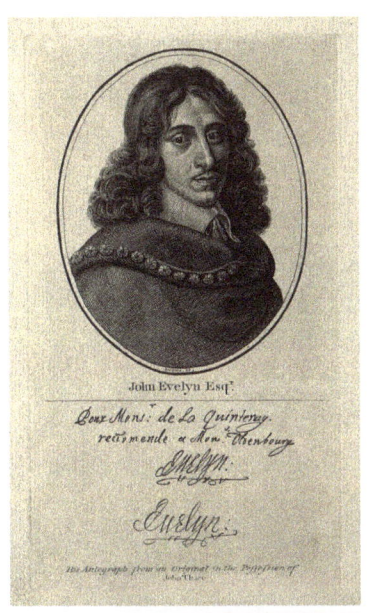

John Evelyn
Wellcome Collection

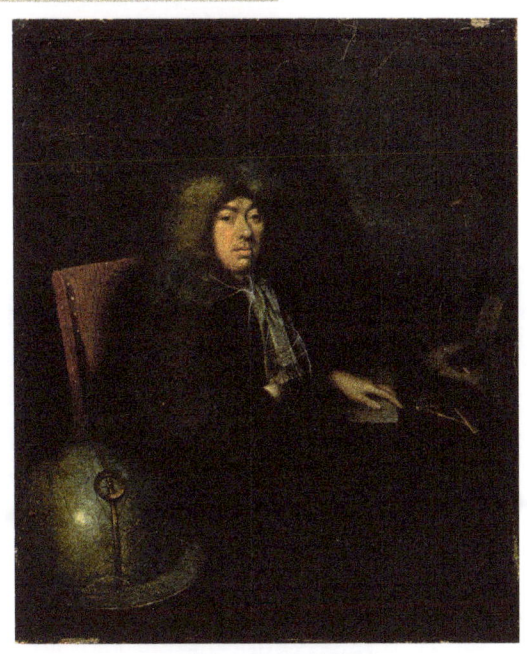

Samuel Pepys
Wellcome Collection

Chapter Five - Quarantine

Quarantine, or isolation, is not a new concept and was understood over 600 years ago to be the most effective way to contain and manage disease.

The Adriatic port of Ragusa (modern day Dubrovnik) was the first to pass mandatory legislation on July 27 1377 forbidding sailing vessels from entering their port, if arriving from plague infested areas. They were ordered to spend a month in Mrkan or the town of Cavtat for disinfection and screening. [1]

The word quarantine is derived from the Italian *'quaranta giorni'* or forty day period, which had symbolic and religious significance for the medieval Christians, following Judeo-Christian tradition. Forty days was a time for ritual purification. The flood lasted forty days and nights and Jesus fasted in the wilderness for forty days. He appeared to his disciples forty days after the crucifixion. After childbirth the lying in period was typically forty days.

Quarantine also has another purpose besides managing and attempting containment. It may restore or assist in the achievement of a sense of order. Pandemics can result in panic, societal breakdown or mass complacency. Confident and consistent decision making is vital to provide the public with a sense of security and trust in those set in authority.

Quarantine includes provision for those infected, in order to separate them from healthy communities and provide care and treatment to attempt recovery. Plague hospitals were set up after the leper houses were no longer required. The first reported plague hospital was set up at Mljet, which became known as a 'lazaretto', a corruption of the word 'Nazaretto' Venice built its first permanent plague hospital on a lagoon island and called it *'Santa Maria di Nazareth'*. [2]

At the same time as the Royal College of Physicians was set up in 1518, quarantine was attempted in London. This was on the orders of Cardinal Wolsey, due to an outbreak of plague. Wolsey sought advice from the learned physician Thomas Linacre, who had benefited from studying medicine in Padua. [3]

Outbreaks of the plague swept across the world in waves, but in 1575 Venice suffered a great outbreak of the plague, leaving at least a third of their population dead. It was at a time of religious unrest between the Jewish quarter and the Catholics in the City, (see Shakespeare play Merchant of Venice), so it was believed that God was exacting his vengeance on the City. The dead and dying were taken by boat to the lagoon island of Lazarretto Vecchio. This site was used between 1403 – 1630. The richer merchants of Venice however were transported to the Lazerreto

Nuovo and buried in shallow graves. The latter was used from 1468.

It is debatable how effective quarantine actually was, just as it is controversial today to gauge how effective lockdowns have been in containment of infection. Quarantine success requires compliance and trust in those in authority. There were riots in London recorded as the poor rebelled against the restrictions, little different from the protests we have seen over recent times. An example was at The Ship Tavern, Holborn, when the landlord was ordered to 'shut up' his ale house. Orders were released by the Lord Mayor barring second hand trade, as it was understood that recycled bedding and clothing could pass on the disease. Quarantine and lockdown appear to flatten the incidence of disease, but infection rates seem to rise again once quarantine measures are relaxed.

The streets became deadly quiet and the playhouses were boarded up

'To play in plagetime is to increase the plage by infection: to play out of plagetime is to draw the plage by offendinges of God upon occasion of such playes.' [4].

John Evelyn similarly observed 'no rattling coaches, no prancing horses, no *calling in customers, and no offering wares.'* [5].

Chapter Six - Pavage and sanitation – the changing urban environment.

As early as 1268 the Crown made at least fifty-nine awards of pavage (paving streets) up until 1308, as it was understood that dirt was a prime convector of distemper and contagion. By the end of the fourteenth century everyone, except the lowest illiterate in society, knew about the threat of miasmic air. Paving was important as it enabled refuse collectors to clear the streets. Communal dumps were set up, organised by the scavengers, rakers and rag and bone men. Certain prohibitions were brought in, for example the heaping of dung was prohibited in York in 1301 [1]

A focus of disease was seen to stem from the slaughter houses, or the shambles, where blood and offal remains were thrown out into the streets. Laystalls, or the ground where cattle were herded, got filled up with cattle dung and were seen as hotbeds of infection. So these areas were targeted by the rakers too. Markets in towns and cities could endanger the whole community [2].

Stow and others disapproved of the urban growth in London in the sixteenth century [3]. Elizabeth I was not happy to allow uncontrolled urban growth during her reign. In 1580 she issued a proclamation prohibiting new house building within three miles of any London gate. Despite this edict being reissued in 1593 and 1602, it made little difference, until the Great Fire of 1666 when it was possible for redesign. [4].

Champion focuses on the social context for disease [5], arguing that the standard of environmental living determined the extent and type of mortality experienced.

Rivers were also associated with disease and death. [6] The River Fleet in London was renowned for the stench along its course.

> *'in every parish along the Fleet, the plague stayed and destroyed.' [7]*

This then led onto the rise of squalor and crime. [8]. Cholera outbreaks hit the people living nearest the rivers the most [9] The increasing number of epidemics resulted in the creation of eight regional boards of Commissioners of Sewers in 1531. [10] Sadly the Commissioners did not have the foresight to build new sewers, but only repaired existing ones. Eventually the rivers were covered over.

Little changed over the following years until the Victorian era. By the eighteenth century it became the legal duty of every householder to pave the street up to the centre line of the street in front of his house [11]. However this resulted in bumps and holes along a patchy street. Added to this was the disruption caused by the water companies, the only utility company by the seventeenth century. They laid wooden pipes, which were constantly under repair. By 1760 a clean-up campaign was launched, with a tax raised to cover the cost. Streets were cambered, with a gutter each side. [12]. Commissioners were introduced to regulate public utilities, including the roads and street lighting.

Elm trees were planted round the streets and squares, as elm gave the best shade and endured coal smoke, retaining its leaves until autumn. The Victorians were more in favour of plane trees, resulting in the mix of species we see today.

In the late nineteenth century public bath houses were built for the urban working classes. By the beginning of the twentieth century most new houses had running water and toilets, although poverty and deprivation was rife with slum dwellings. [13]

The evidence shows that later medieval England did not trail behind her European neighbours, but endeavoured to advance sanitary regulation, with an understanding that poor sanitation increased contagion [14]

Chapter Seven – Events leading up to 1665

664 AD is the recorded date for the first pestilential outbreak in Britain, [1] as testified by Beda in his *'Ecclesiastical History'* [2]. The common name for the plague was *pestis, pestilential* or *magna mortalitas.* It was also known as the *'botch'*, because of the botches or swellings that appeared over the body and in particular under the armpits.

The earliest hospitals were the leper hospitals. Nearly half the number of English hospitals founded were allied to the monasteries. One of the most famous is that built by Matilda, wife to Henry I. Built in 1101, it was situated in St Giles in the Fields, London. It had a capacity to care for up to forty lepers. Leprosy was an indeterminate diagnosis, [3] so those cared for might have been suffering a range of illnesses. More than twenty-six hospitals were founded by Royalty between 1118 – 1251 AD. Travellers at this time would be greeted by the hospitium of these places [4]. The next hospitals built were more like alms-houses; to care for the poor and destitute. The two most famous are St Bartholomew's and St Thomas's in London. St. Bartholomew's Hospital was founded in 1123 in the City and St. Thomas's was built in 1170, attached to St. Mary Overie in

Southwark. This is now Southwark Cathedral. After the Reformation Henry VIII and his son Edward VI rebuilt and improved these hospitals. St. Bartholomew's was restored in 1548 and St. Thomas's in 1553 by Edward VI. At this time Christ's hospital and Bridewell were erected and Bethlehem Hospital (Bedlam) for the insane. 'Lock' hospitals were eventually set up in the disused leper hospitals, when leprosy was no longer prevalent. [5]. They cared for those with venereal diseases like syphilis, which were very prevalent in Tudor society. By the eighteenth century hospitals were being built, through private benevolence and philanthropy. Westminster hospital is noted to be the first provided through subscription, followed by hospitals like Guys and the Middlesex. A smallpox hospital was built in 1746 on the Kings Cross site in response to the rising number of smallpox cases.

Pest houses were being used in a very much ad hoc way before 1665. There were originally only two in London, situated in Old Street and Tothill Fields. Eventually three more were erected to help cope with the massive extent of infection during the year of 1665.

Following the introduction of quarantine measures in 1518, Cardinal Wolsey declared that infected houses had to hang a bundle of straw outside their houses for forty days, to warn others of the risk. The straw had to be hung on a pole ten foot long, to ensure visibility. If anyone from an infected house ventured outside they had to carry a rod four feet long, in order to be identified and avoided.

Charles Creighton includes the full text -

'35 Hen. VIII. A precept issued to the aldermen:—that they should cause their beadles to set the sign of the cross on every house which should be afflicted with the plague, and there continue for forty days'

'That no person who was able to live by himself, and should be afflicted with the plague, should go abroad or into any company for one month after his sickness, and that all others who could not live without their daily labour should as much as in them lay refrain from going abroad, and should for forty days after and continually carry a white rod in their hand, two foot long:

'That every person whose house had been infected should, after a visitation, carry all the straw and in the night privately into the fields and burn; they should also carry clothes of the infected in the fields to be cured:

'That no housekeeper should put any person diseased out of his house into the street or other place unless they provided housing for them in some other house:

'That all persons having any dogs in their

houses other than hounds, spaniels or mastiffs, necessary for the custody or safe keeping of their houses, should forthwith convey them out of the city, or cause them to be killed and carried out of the city and buried at the common laystall:

'That such as kept hounds, spaniels, or mastiffs should not suffer them to go abroad, but closely confine them:

'That the churchwardens of every parish should employ somebody to keep out all common beggars out of churches on holy days, and to cause them to remain without doors:

'That all the streets, lanes, etc. within the wards should be cleansed:

'That the aldermen should cause this precept to be read in the churches.' [6]

By 1521 parishioners had to put a red St Anthony's cross on their door, or Tau cross as it was known, as it resembled the Greek letter tau. [7]. In 1543 the cross had to remain on the front of the house for forty days and those that left their houses had to carry a white rod, now two foot long. Four years later in 1547 regulations had changed yet again and the crosses had to be painted blue. All the marked houses were checked by the Parish Clerks and Justices of the Peace.

By 1570, in the reign of Elizabeth I quarantine measures were reduced by half to twenty days. It is not documented why changes in quarantine were made, so one can only surmise that from observations it was believed that forty day quarantine was unnecessary and too long. We can see the similarities today where self-isolation periods for those infected and in contact with those with Covid 19 have been changeable.

By 1574 a Royal Decree was issued ordering that houses infected with plague had to write *'Lord have mercy upon us'* on their doors. Also at this time women searchers were employed to search out infection in the homes. They were paid the princely sum of three pence for each examination. Two searchers entered at a time and were regulated by the Parish, to avoid unsavoury characters exploiting their position.

By 1582 the white rods were replaced with red rods and in 1592 red crosses had to be painted on the doors.

Two years following there was the first attempt to provide a Pest House in London, based on Milan's Lazerreto di San Gregorio,which had been erected in 1488.

Red rods were now increased to three foot long and the 'shutting up' system was introduced. The inhabitants of infected houses were strictly monitored leaving their homes and rarely were permitted out.

Two discreet matrons within every parish

who shall be sworn truly to search the body of every such person as shall happen to die within the same parish, of their reporting to the Clerk of the Parish [8], *and of the clerk making report and certificate to the wardens of the Parish Clerks, who would send the weekly certificate for all the parishes to the Mayor, and he to the Minister of State. That was said to be 'according to the order in that behalf heretofore provided'*

It is probable, therefore, that the searchers became an institution as early as the plague of 1563, or, at all events, at the beginning of the plague-period of 1578-83. [9]

Simon Kellwaye in 1592 wrote that which

'Teacheth what orders magistrates and rulers of Citties and townes shoulde cause to be observed.

1. First to command that no stinking doonghills be suffered neere the Cittie.

2. Every evening and morning in the hot weather to cause colde water to be cast in the streetes, especially where the infection is, and every day to cause the streets to be kept cleane and sweete, and clensed from all filthie thinges which lye in the same.

3. And whereas the infection is entred, there to cause fires to be made in the streetes every morning and evening, and if some frankincense, pitch or some other sweet thing be burnt therein it will be much the better.

4. Suffer not any dogs, cattes, or pigs to run about the streets, for they are very dangerous, and apt to carry the infection from place to place.

5. Command that the excrements and filthy things which are voided from the infected places be not cast into the streets, or rivers which are daily in use to make drink or dress meat.

6. That no Chirurgions, or barbers, which use to let blood, do cast the same into the streets or rivers.

7. That no vautes or previes be then emptied, for it is a most dangerous thing.

8. That all Inholders do every day make clean their stables, and cause the doong and filth therein to be carryed away out of the Cittie; for, by suffering it in their houses, as some do use to do, a whole week or fortnight, it doth so putrifie that when it is removed, there is such a stinking savour and unwholesome smell, as is able to infect the whole street where it is.

9. To command that no hemp or flax be kept in water neere the Cittie or towne, for that will cause a very dangerous and infectious savour.

10. To have a speciall care that good and wholesome victuals and corne be solde in the markets, and so to provide that no want thereof be in the Cittie, and for such as have not wherewithall to buy necessary food, that there to extend their charitable and goodly devotion; for there is nothing that will more encrease the plague than want and scarcity of necessary food.

11. To command that all those which do visit and attend the sick, as also all those which have the sickness on them, and do walk abroad: that they do carry something in their hands, thereby to be known from other people.

Lastly, if the infection be in but few places, there to keep all the people in their houses, all necessaries being brought to them. When the plague is staid, then to cause all the clothes, bedding, and other such things as were used about the sick to be burned, although at the charge of the rest of the inhabitants you buy them all new.' [10]

As the population grew, so did the death rate from contagion. Efforts were then taken to control infections, but it is dubious how effective their restraining practices actually were. The Privy Council informed the Lord Mayor that the incidence of disease was accelerating to unacceptable levels. Again comparisons can be made with our most recent pandemic, where the R rate, or reproduction rate of Sars co-V was monitored.

A degree of classification of diseases did not begin until 1519, with the first London Bill of Mortality. The Bills were more explanatory from 1555, when information was included about what the disease was and where it occurred. It is difficult to be clear exactly what diseases were prevalent at certain periods, as measles, flu and smallpox were widespread at the same time as the plague. The earliest reference to smallpox is made in 1514/18 when it is written that *'pokes and mezils and the great sickness'* were present in England [11]. Interestingly, smallpox was not considered particularly virulent in the sixteenth century and it was only in the seventeenth century that smallpox became more feared. Elizabeth I suffered smallpox in 1562, wrapping herself in red cloth, which was thought to withdraw the disease from the body. She survived, but was left with unsightly facial scarring. From this time on she used white lead make up which may have ultimately led to her demise from lead poisoning in 1603.

Comparing the weekly Bills of Mortality for smallpox around the time of the last Great Plague of 1665, we see that the incidence is low

in comparison to the plague, which was killing Londoners in their thousands.
Deaths in London 1664: 1233
Deaths in London 1665: 655
Deaths in London 1666: 38 [12]

Mortality in London from the plague was greatest in 1603, 1625 and 1665, although there were regular outbreaks in frequent intervals across the whole of the country. The plague of 1603 coincided with the death of Elizabeth I and the accession of James I. The second main outbreak in 1625 coincided with the accession of Charles I. It was believed that plague hit at these times as a result of the sins over the previous reign. A new Monarch gave them the opportunity to repent of their previous sins [13].

From the middle of the seventeenth century to the middle of the nineteenth century, the Bills of Mortality were printed and issued every Thursday. By 1665 there were 140 parishes in London, which produced weekly Bills of Mortality. [14]

	Estimated population	Total deaths	Plague deaths	Highest mortality in a week	Worst week	
1603	250,000	42,940	33,347	3385	25 Aug.-1 Sept.
1625	320,000	63,001	41,313	5205	11-18 Aug.
1665	460,000	97,306	68,596	8297	12-19 Sept.

Defoe's description of the plague year is the most revealing account we have of 1665, but other writings of interest are those of William Boghurst (1630-1685), a young apothecary, who was practising his trade at the White Hart, Drury Lane, in St Giles in the Fields. He was treating many people with the plague and advertised that he could treat with

'water, a lozenge, and an electuary, as well as an antidote, at 8d an ounce' [15].

An electuary is a mix of powdered herbs and honey. After his death, his works were initially in the hands of Sir Hans Sloane, but now his manuscripts are in the British Museum, London [16]

Dr Nathaniel Hodges was two years older than Boghurst and he wrote two learned treatises on the plague. The most famous is *Loimologia, or a Historical Account of the Plague in London,* which was published in 1672. He realised that treatments for the common people were what was needed primarily and the physician needed to have a cheerful disposition [17]. He stayed in London during the plague and worked tirelessly helping the sick, who either visited his practice, or he visited patients at home. He swore by the effectiveness of sack against plague and drank this every evening. Sack was similar to sherry. He realised that the best strategy was to remove the sick as soon as possible from their homes, in order to remove the risk of spread to the rest of the household. He had poor regard for the nurses who he described as

'wretches, out of greediness to plunder the dead, would strangle their patients and charge it to the distemper in their throats' [18].

He questioned the efficacy of classical cures and based his practice more on empirical observation.

Daniel Defoe was only aged four in 1665, but in 1722 at the age of sixty-one he completed writing the notes left from his Uncle Henry Foe. He records how the plague spread from parish to parish, starting in the west in St Giles and moving east. In 1663 plague was ravaging Holland. Charles II stopped all trade and eventually went to war with Holland. A single death was recorded in Long Acre in December 1664 and no attention was paid to it. There were nearly half a million inhabitants in London by 1665, so a single death from plague of distemper did not cause any concern. However the numbers soared the following year with two thirds of the population fleeing into the country. The nonconformist preacher Thomas Vincent (1634 – 1678) remarked

'death riding triumphantly on his pale horse through our streets' [19]

Vincent wrote the lengthy sermon titled '*God's terrible voice in the City*' claiming that the plague had hit the country as a result of God's wrath on account of their sins and acts of debauchery. [20]. William Petty, an eminent statistician devised a rule of thumb that when the weekly death toll from the plague reached a hundred, it triggered an exodus from the City. It was predominantly only the poor who were left, apart from those who were prepared to risk their lives and wished to protect their livelihoods, like Henry Foe. Charles II moved out to Salisbury and then to Oxford, but gave £1000 from his purse every week to support the City

It was a dilemma for physicians and clergy alike – should they stay and run the risk of dying from the plague, or should they flee into the country so that they could care for the survivors once the plague had abated? It was a difficult choice for many. With the loss of clergy and physicians the market opened up to apothecaries with their various pills and potions and the void in physic led to an increase in the practice of quackery.

Trade was severely affected during the plague years. Ships, especially from Holland, were held at the quarantine station. The river was seen as an escape and refuge from the plague [21]. Pepys tells us that two thirds of shops and trades shut in the Seething Lane area within two months of the Great Plague [22]. The only businesses that thrived were the apothecaries, quacks, butchers, cooks and coffin makers. Pepys bravely was the only naval administrator to remain at the Navy Office. [23]. The Exchequer had moved away to the old Tudor Palace of Nonsuch, where Pepys had to make the perilous journey quite regularly. [24] Surprisingly Pepys found the plague year one of his happiest and busiest, as he was able to lead effectively a bachelor existence, visiting mistresses as he pleased. [25].

The Lord Mayor, Sir John Lawrence, with the Justices of the Peace, administered relief across the parishes. John Lawrence lived at the Guildhall and spoke with the parishioners from his gallery in the Great Hall. He knew that it would be safer to practise social distancing, even at this time.

The burning of fires, releasing sulphur, which initially was thought to expel the infection from the air, was discontinued by the autumn of 1665. This was because of heavy rains in the autumn, differences in medical opinion as to whether coal or wood fires were the most effective and finally because of the popular perception that the practice had no effect on quelling the plague.

Most of the provincial outbreaks in 1665 were due to the transmission of the plague from London. The story of the small village of Eyam in Derbyshire will be described in the following chapter.

The history of plague in England ends with a report of death at Rotherhithe in east London in 1679.

Why did the plague end quite so abruptly and why didn't it die down gradually? It is thought that plague is principally a disease of commerce and with the closure of trade routes from the Levant and Asia, the infection abated.

However, even today there are outbreaks of plague. About 3000 cases a year are reported worldwide [26]

Chapter Eight - The Story of Eyam

At the time of the plague Eyam was a small village near Chesterfield, with 350 inhabitants. It seemed to be a million miles away from London, which was 160 miles to the south. The incumbent Rector Reverend William Mompesson had only recently taken up his post. He was twenty-seven years old, with a wife and two small children. There was no resident doctor in the village.

On the third of September 1665 a box arrived from London for the tailor Edward Cooper. He instructed his servant George Vicars to open it. He hung the damp cloth sent from London out to dry. Tragically there were fleas infected with the plague in the cloth.

The nature of the disease has been challenged in recent times, with some suggesting the disease was typhus, anthrax or measles, [1] but following detailed analysis the only possible explanation is that it was bubonic plague.

A parish register was compiled by a later Rector, Joseph Hunt, including the years 1630 – 1700. This register is now stored with the Derbyshire Record Society [2] Analysis concludes that there was at least 75 per cent transmission from person to person [3] This evidence has resulted in mathematical modelling of transmission [4].

There have been debates about the ethics and principles of quarantine, [5] but inadvertently the inhabitants of Eyam did the right thing by containing the spread [6].

One by one the villagers died as the infection rampaged from home to home. The village looked to the Church for guidance. As Mompesson was relatively new the villagers called upon the previous Rector to return. This was the Reverend Thomas Stanley, who had been ejected for his nonconformist views in 1662. However, he had been well liked and trusted in the village, so they sought his wisdom as to how to manage the contagion.

Mompesson and Stanley discussed how they could best contain the infection and called the whole village together. They instructed the village to –

- Meet for Sunday services outside and spaced apart in Cuckold Delft, a field nearby.
- That no –one must leave the village boundary
- Food and provisions would be supplied by the neighbouring village Stoney Middleton and from the Earl of Devonshire, who lived at Chatsworth.

In the spring of 1666, long after it had abated in London, the villagers of Eyam witnessed the full force of the disease.

The Rector's wife gave pastoral care to many and sadly on the 25th August 1666 while walking on the hills with William she remarked about the sweet smelling air. This was a typical sign of infection and she died three days later. Every year in Eyam the village lay red roses on her tomb, in remembrance of her goodness and selflessness.

Suddenly in the October of 1666 the plague ran its course.

In total seventy-six households were infected and 259 buried. The people were buried in shallow graves, allowing emanations of plague to rise from the soil and poison the whole valley.

A few wealthy households fled and it is not believed that they spread it to other communities. Afterwards Mompesson moved out to Eakring in Nottingham and eventually remarried. Mompesson held the best motives, but there was no scientific basis for his and Thomas Stanley's decision. In effect the whole village was 'shut up' and many died. It has been argued that it would have been better to isolate the initial household that was infected and minimise the risk of others catching the plague? [7]

The story illustrates the struggle between science and religion, at a time when society was at the cusp of the modern world. Geraldine Brooks, war correspondent has brought the story to life in her fictional account of that fateful year. [8]

The next chapter explains the coordinated system that Charles II set in place, which centred round the concept of self-isolation and containment using a network of Pest Houses.

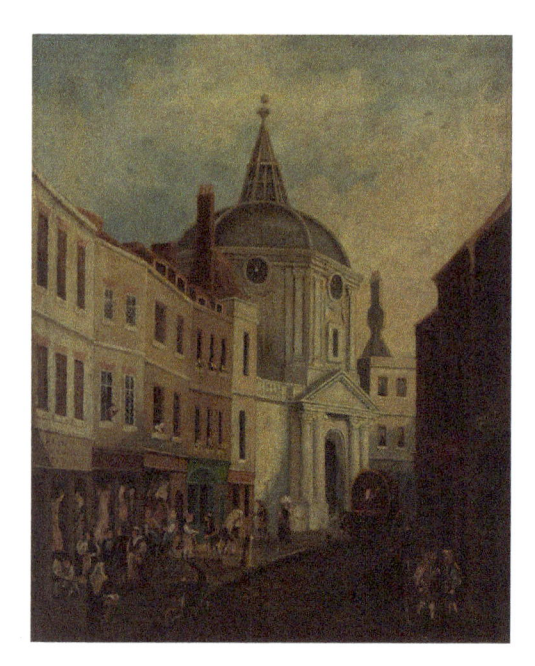

Royal College of Physicians, Warwick Lane, London
Wellcome Collection

Orders for the Plague
Look and Learn

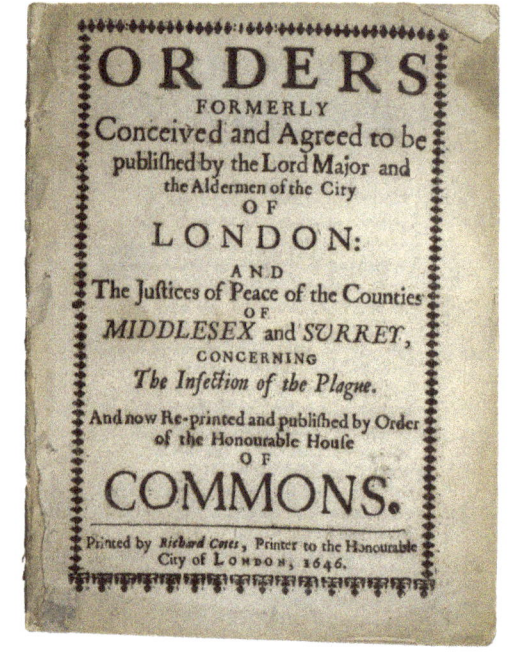

The Kings
Medicine
1665
Look and Learn

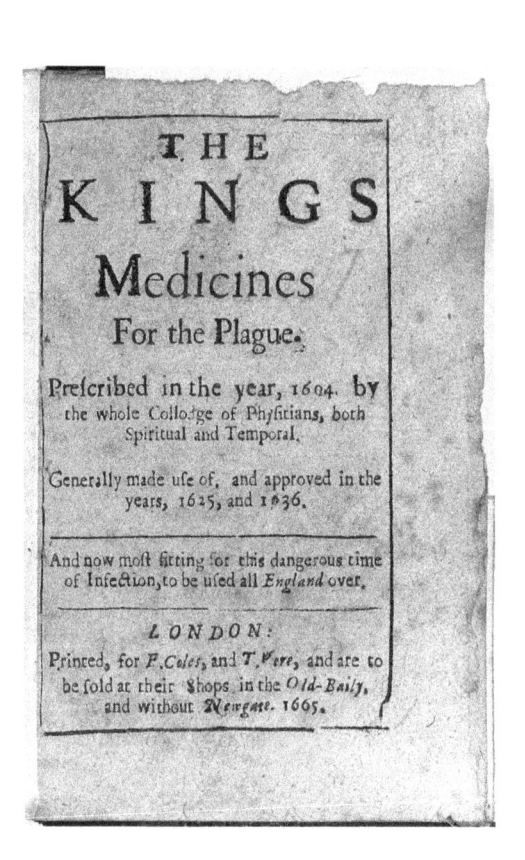

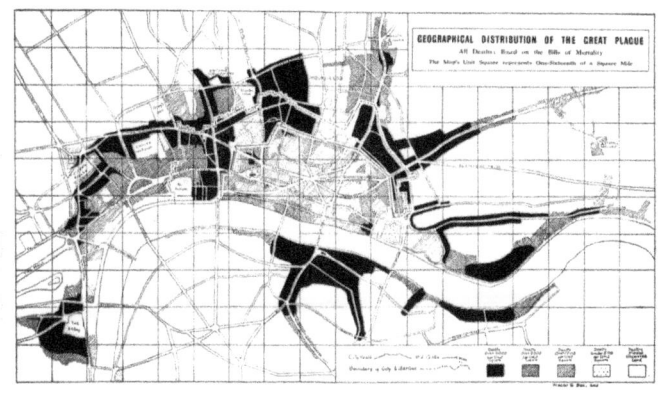

THE
KINGS
Medicines
For the Plague.

Prescribed in the year, 1604, by the whole Colledge of Physitians, both Spiritual and Temporal.

Generally made use of, and approved in the years, 1625, and 1636.

And now most fitting for this dangerous time of Infection, to be used all *England* over.

LONDON:
Printed, for F. Coles, and T. Vere, and are to be sold at their Shops in the *Old-Baily*, and without *Newgate*. 1665.

Geographical distribution of the Great Plague
Look and Learn

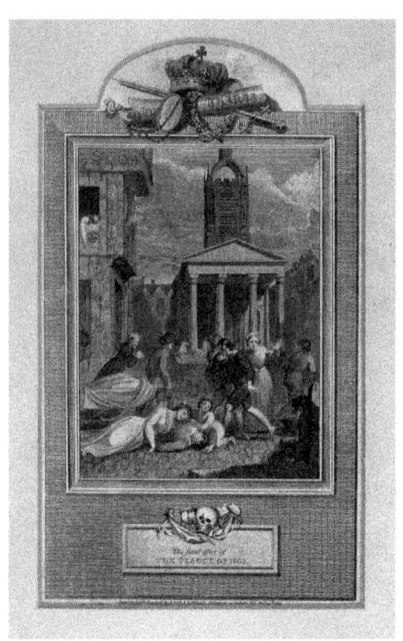

The Plague of 1665
Look and Learn

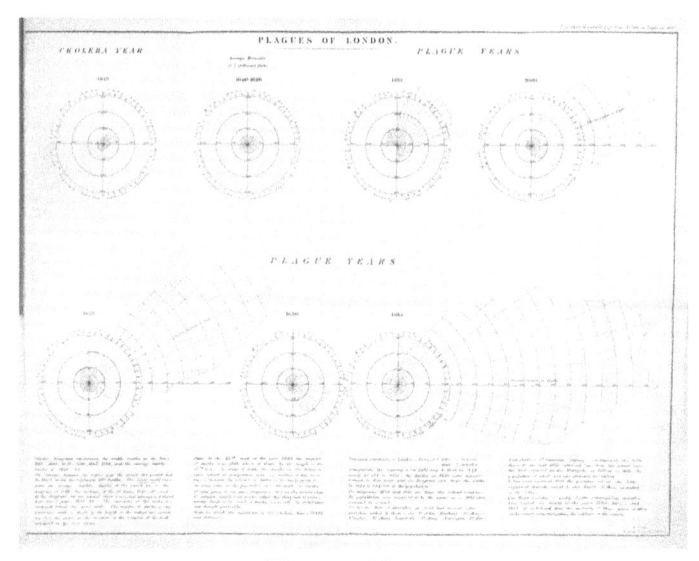

Plague Years
Look and Learn

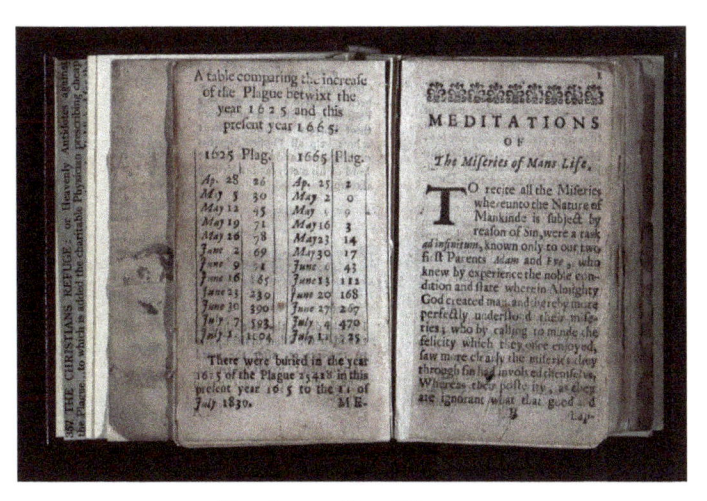

Book on the Plague
Look and Learn

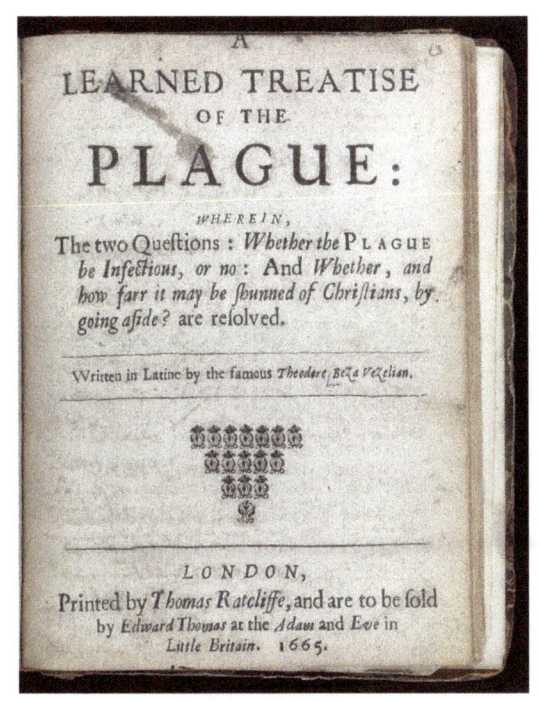

Book continued
Look and Learn

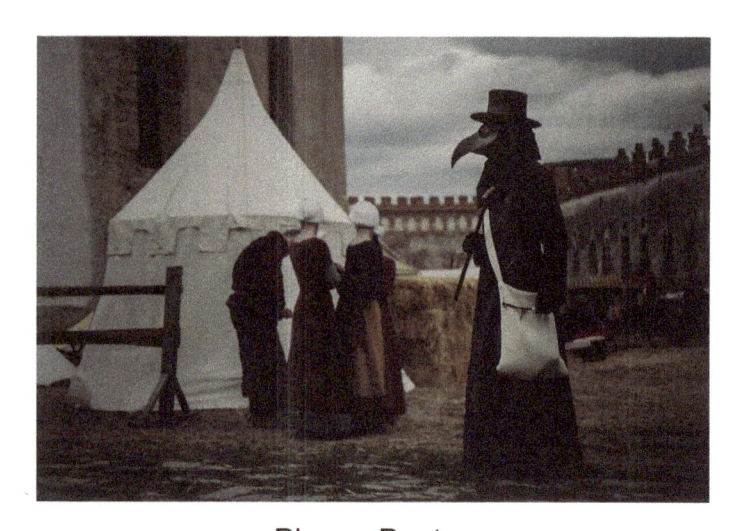

Plague Doctor
Shutterstock

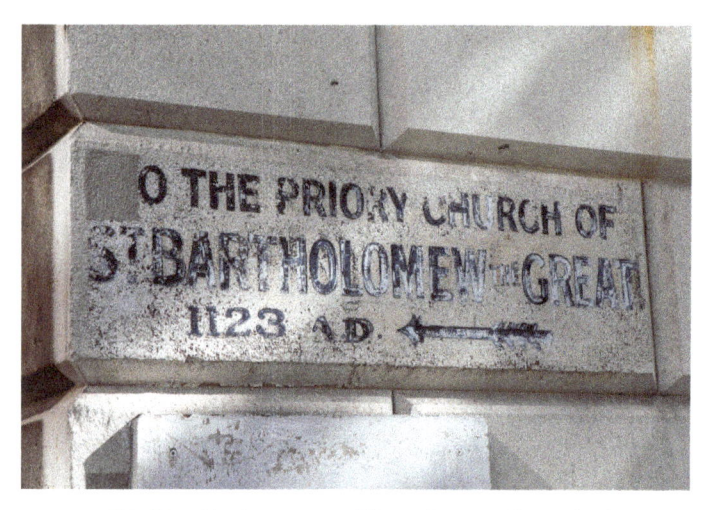

St. Bartholomews The Great Hospital
Shutterstock

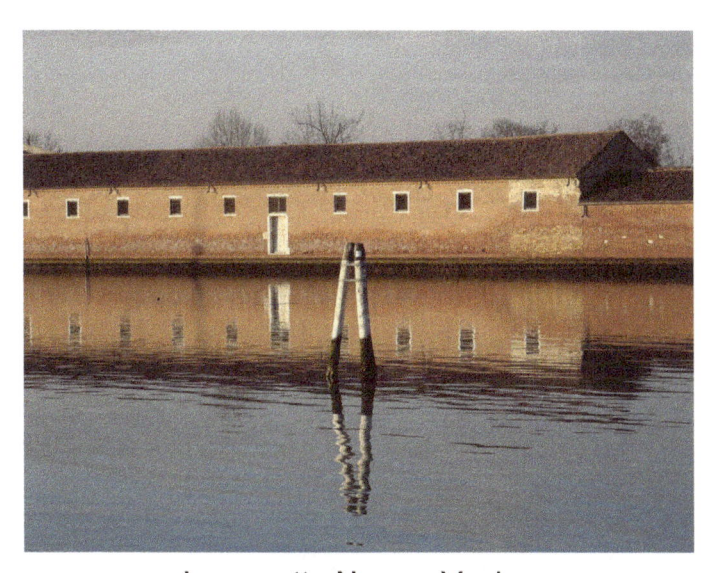

Lazzeretto Nuovo, Venice
Shutterstock

Burying the dead
Shutterstock

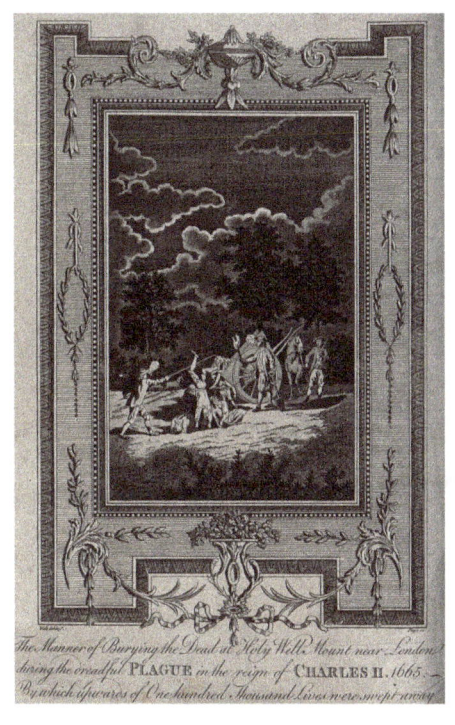

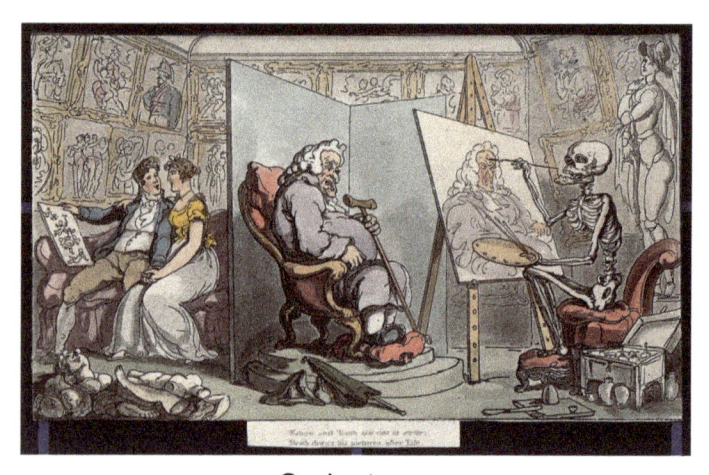

Caricatures
Wellcome Collection

Chapter nine - The pest house system

How did it all start in 1665?

We have a number of diarists to thank for providing information about the day to day conditions of 1665. Defoe, Boghurst and Pepys have already been mentioned. Another diarist, John Allin, lived close by to Samuel Pepys in St.Olave's, He believed that people had to repent, to rid themselves of the distemper. Pardon of sin was to him the best cordial [1]. In addition to his deeply held views, he was a firm parachelist. He believed wholeheartedly in alchemy, suggesting the use of 'angell gold' [2]

Admiral Lord Sandwich, commanding in Portsmouth, reported a strange new star in the west at the beginning of 1665. Charles II was fascinated by the occult and astrology and waited to see this comet for himself. It was seen the most clearly from Tower Hill. The people believed it was a sign of impending doom. [3] A second comet appeared, bigger and brighter than the first in March and resulted in widespread trepidation. [4]

London became so overcrowded after the Restoration in 1660, that the City could not reasonably contain the numbers. [5]. Charles II promoted both economy and trade, with craftsmen moving into London from all over the country and from Europe. [6]. John Graunt (1620-1674), a member of the Royal Society and statistician in 1665 stated that

> *'the parishes are now grown madly disproportionable… the old streets are unfit for the present frequency of coaches.'* [7]

Graunt produced weekly Bills of Mortality, detailing the specific causes of death in more than 130 parishes and was one of the first demographers. These Bills could be read by anyone paying four shillings a year.

Not only did the country endure the terrible suffering and death from plague, but Britain had declared war with Holland in February 1665, which continued during this period.

The plague outbreak started quietly, with several competing stories as to its origin. As there was no understanding of disease causation, marginal groups were generally blamed for outbreaks of epidemics [8]. One report is of an isolated case of two Frenchman becoming ill in Long Acre, near Drury Lane. Others blame a Mary Ramsey who had travelled from the West Country carrying cloth. However the first recorded death is that of a young servant who died in the home of Dr Nathaniel Rogers over the Christmas of 1664. [9]. It's conceivable that when the cases were few in number that people concealed the infection, as they knew they would have to isolate. It was also easy to confuse symptoms as there were many infections, for example scurvy, which was also prevalent at the time.

In 1665 the death toll rose inexorably; in London alone the number recorded was 68,596, although the rate was likely to be much higher. It is actually believed that 100,000 or a quarter of the population of London succumbed to the plague. Anabaptists, Quakers and Jews would have nothing to do with the Protestant Church, as they believed it violated their own faith, and they did not record their own deaths. Also, many paupers were just thrown into plague pits.

As stated before, it was the poor who were left to bear the brunt of the contagion. The wealthy had options, for example Pepys sent his wife to Greenwich and King Charles II left the City and went to Salisbury and from there onwards to Oxford. Ben Johnson's play '*The Alchemist*' written in 1610 before the Great Plague, illustrates in a comical way the events that might occur when a gentleman flees the plague and leaves his house under the sole charge of a servant. [10]

Parishes were ordered to kill their cats and dogs; as a result 40,000 dogs and 200,000 cats were destroyed in London, as they were thought to be carriers of the fleas. In fact it would have been far more effective to have left the cats to control the rat population. Those who killed the animals were rewarded with two pence per dead animal.

Bubonic plague, with the accompanying

characteristic swellings or buboes was the type of plague spreading fast through the population. On a positive note it is said that 20 to 30 per cent of those who fell ill survived. Lancing, or the bursting of buboes, seemed to have aided recovery, possibly as it enabled the poisonous exudate to drain away.

The hospitals would not admit plague victims, as the hospital authorities realised the plague would kill both patients and staff. [11] At the time St.Bartholomews had fifteen nursing sisters, assisted by 'helpers', sometimes called nurses. There were 200-300 beds. [12] The Matron, Margaret Blague, remained in her post during the plague and ministered to the poor in the street, taking them broth and caudles. [13] She was the widow of a barber-surgeon and was matron for thirty-two years, until her death in 1675. [14]

'Shutting up' was still the common practice, but the King had ordered every parish to designate a place of safety and care – the Pest House – overseen by the Parish Clerks and Justices of the Peace. It was at this point in history that government became more involved in public health measures. [15] People were recognising that solely 'shutting up' was wrong for moral and economic reasons. James Bamford, vicar of St.Olaves, Southwark viewed the custom as 'a bloudy error.' [16]

Morally, could it be right to shut up healthy residents of plague infected houses, or should they have the chance to work and survive? If all the economically active died, there would be a huge impact on the country, as befell England in 1348.

Boghurst did not mince his words in his condemnation of the 'shutting up' process. He called it murder. [17] Dr Hodges also criticised the 'shutting up' method for isolating people inside their homes, with no assistance provided. [18]

A regulated system evolved in 1665 and resulted in a new planned system of health protection. An Order was implemented from July 1st 1665. [19]

Defoe outlines the various designated Parish roles:

The Lord Mayor, John Lawrence,

'appointed physicians and surgeons for relief of the diseased poor. He ordered the College of Physicians to publish directions for cheap remedies for the poor.'

Examiners were appointed in every Parish. They held their post for at least two months and their responsibility was to check which houses in their Parish were infected. If anyone refused to accept this role, then they were put into prison. When they discovered infected houses they had to alert the Constables, whose job it was to 'shut up' the premises. The master of every house was obliged to inform the examiner within two hours of any sign of the plague in his house.

Searchers were always women and had to search houses to establish the exact cause of death. They were vetted by the Parish to check they were of good character and were not allowed to do any other work, because of the risk of spreading disease. As Defoe says

'that no searcher during this time of visitation be permitted to use any employment, or keep any shop or stall, or be employed as a laundress...' [20]

They were paid about four pence for each recorded death. There are mixed reports of the competence and trustworthiness of the searchers.

Watchmen were employed in pairs to literally keep watch. They usually carried halberds, padlocks and keys [21]. Daytime shifts were from six am to ten pm. Night time duty started at ten pm and finished at 6am. If the occupants wanted provisions then the watchmen would arrange this, but would carry the key to the 'shut up' house with them.

Dr Thomas Vincent, a divine who remained in London at the time noted *'it was very dismal to behold the red crosses, and read in great letters 'Lord have mercy upon us' on the doors....and watchmen standing beside them with halberts,'* [22]

Quarantine and shutting up was seen as a punishment, with watchmen and constables involved. It was a militaristic style of enforcement. [23] As a consequence, there are several tales of mishaps and murder, as the healthy people living in a house with an infected member could go insane trying to escape. Defoe tells us that they blew up a watchman with gunpowder [24]

This was a system of enforcement and coercion. Anyone seen in the streets with suppurating sores could be fined five pounds, or be put into prison for forty days. There was a hierarchy in the medical marketplace, with greatest status bestowed on physicians. They enjoyed a university training, learning the classical education based on Galenic theories. Surgeons or chirurgeons qualified through an apprenticeship system. They joined together in the guild of barber-surgeons, which was formed in the fifteenth century. The Fellowship of Surgeons joined the barbers in 1540 and it was not until 1745 that the surgeons finally separated from the barbers. From 1745 to 1800 the College of Surgeons was housed in the Old Bailey. [25] The lowest status was that of the apothecary, who acted on the advice of the physicians, concocting remedies advocated by the physician. The word apothecary is derived from 'apotheca' the name for a place where wine, herbs and spices are stored. [26] They evolved from the Company of Grocers, established in 1428. James I created the Worshipful Society of Apothecaries in 1617 and their hall still stands in Blackfriars. [27]

Chirurgeons were chosen, 'in addition to those that belong to the Pest House and were only allowed to work with the diseased. They worked with the searchers to determine death and its cause. Chirurgeons received twelve pence a body searched, to be paid out of the goods of the party searched, if he be able, or otherwise by the Parish. [28]

The first mention of the plague doctor costume is found in the mid seventeenth century writings, by Charles de Lorme, a royal physician to Louis XIII [29] De Lorme states that the doctor wore a waxed Moroccan goat leather coat, with a tight fitting mask, crystal eye pieces and a long beak filled with aromatic herbs.

Nurses as they were called, were not qualified. Many were old and desperate, working only to avoid starvation. *Nurse Keepers* had to isolate if they had been in an infected house within a twenty-eight day period. Some accounts describe really unscrupulous *nurse keepers*, who would hasten the death of plague victims by strangulation, suffocation or giving cold drinks. Their intent was to be paid as quickly as possible for each case they attended. Most came from the roughest class [30] Pepys believed the nurses abused their position to rob the sick and vulnerable [31] To prevent this kind of abuse a system of regulation was devised by the parish. *Nurse keepers* were monitored and held to account, so the situation improved with this new regulated process. It seems genuine care and compassion was demonstrated as well, particularly in the Pest House. The women who worked as *nurse keepers* were those who had previously endured the plague and were therefore thought to be immune.

Generally, no one could leave an infected house unless it was to be carried to the Pest House. So alongside the prescriptive management with the 'shutting up' system there was the parallel system of removal of the sick to the Parish Pest House. It is said there was so much overcrowding that people walked across beds in the Pest House rather than round them. [32]

Three Justices of the Peace bought land to build new Pest Houses. The City and Westminster had their own Pest House, with three more being erected in Marylebone, Soho Fields and Stepney.

Tumbrels were used to transport the dead bodies, which were two wheeled wagons. Hackney coaches and Sudan chairs were used to transport the sick to the Pest House. Charles I had brought these chairs back from his travels in Spain. Pepys comments

'a nurse appointed to her, who being once absent, the mayde got out at the window and run away… she was found walking over the common … and they got one of the pest coaches to carry her to the pest house' [33]

From Pepys observations here it appears that there could have been a degree of coercion to stay and be isolated in the Pest House. The pest coach was not used again for common use, until they had been aired for six days.

St. Margaret's, Westminster, bought a sedan chair, fitted with a strait jacket, used exclusively to carry plague sufferers to the Westminster Pest

House. Once sick women arrived at the Pest House they were dressed in sack like garments, known as sick dresses.

Rakers and *scavengers* were employed to sweep away the filth from homes and their vicinity. The filth was then carried away to communal dumps. The filth was so bad that people often used pattens, or odd shaped metal platforms, which fitted beneath their shoes. These could be removed when entering a house. [34]. Not only was there filth on the ground, but the flies that filled the noxious air were putrifying the air. William Boghurst remarked that

'there was such a multitude of flyes that they lined the insides of houses' [35]

So where possible the sick were carried away to the parish Pest House, where they would be visited by the *nurse keepers* and physicians. It became increasingly clear that the 'shutting-up' system was inappropriate, inadequate and cruel. There were even stories told that people were maliciously shut-up when they were well, with no signs of symptoms of the plague. At least if people went to the Pest House and were found to be well, they could be released. [36]

All those appointed to various roles by the parish were required to carry wooden rods whilst on their business, in order to be readily identifiable. In order to finance the system of relief and regulation a poor relief rate was levied of a few pence per household. [37]

However, Defoe laments the fact that London lacked the capacity to cope with the numbers that needed care in Pest Houses. He remarks that it was a great mistake that only two Pest Houses were initially available in London. One near Bunhill Fields could accommodate 200-300 people and was by far the largest. The other one was situated in Westminster in Tothill Fields.

It seems from Defoe's account, which as we know was taken from the daily writings of his Uncle Henry Foe living through it, that staying in the Pest House really saved many. As Defoe states

'for very many were sent out again whole; and very good physicians were appointed' [38]

He goes on to say that the principal occupants of the Pest House were servants who had caught the plague from making errands for the family. Defoe gives us the number who actually died at these Pest Houses. 156 were buried at the City Pest House and 159 at Westminster Pest House. However, the fate for those left on their own without their maids and manservants could be contrary to the experience of those carried swiftly to the Pest Houses, where they were given food, warmth and care.

Large quantities of coal was burnt to keep the sick warm, even in the height of summer. This was done on the advice of the physician. The other reason why fires were lit and in some houses they were burning almost continuously, was to sweeten and purge the air.

The plight for pregnant women was highlighted by Boghurst [39]. He estimated that only two per cent of women survived, or if they survived they suffered a stillborn or miscarriages. Midwives were reluctant to deliver infected women, but if they were looked after it was generally by ignorant untrained women.

The mental and emotional effects of the plague can be understated. Nearly half of the victims went mad prior to death. The pain was so intense that people were known to apply burning embers to their body. Suicides also were common, as the pain was so unbearable.

The King issued Orders for the Prevention of the Plague in 1666 [40]

The strict regulations that had to be followed did not end at death. Burials took place under the auspices of the parish buriers, as they were called [41]. Burials had to take place in the hours of darkness, which became a challenge to comply with in the summer months, when the nights were short. Gatherings at funerals were strictly limited to six [42]. This was difficult to enforce as people wanted to be with their loved ones to say goodbye.

Travel was permissible initially, but by June 1665, Certificates of Health were required in order to travel. These were issued in London by the Lord Mayor, Sir John Lawrence. Those who attempted to flout the rules were often discovered and fined, and taken back into the city walls.

From London the plague spread out to the suburbs via trade routes and Braintree, Colchester and Norwich were particularly affected. One thousand or a third of the population died of the plague in Braintree. Provisions were left for them in a field outside Rayne. Colchester was hit hardest, with half of their population decimated. Nearly five thousand died there. [43].There were two Pest Houses in Colchester, at St. Mary's and Mile End. [44]. The other main affected areas recorded were Portsmouth, Southampton, Sunderland and Newcastle. [45]

The plague had a big impact on the economy and livelihood of many. In fact it was the middle classes who suffered the most, the merchants and entrepreneurs who had never received poor relief were now dependant on the parish for help. Vendors of perishable goods were hit hardest, as they lost income from reduced sales and spoilage of their produce. The very poor would already exist on poor relief, which was collected within each Parish, so their financial situation did not change markedly. [46]. Parallels can be drawn to the present day and will be discussed later.

Chapter Ten - Pest Houses demolished in England.

The Pest House system was the successor to the lazaretto or leper house. Some of the early Pest Houses across the country were disused leper houses. The first leper or lobe house was erected in York in 936 AD. [1]. Leprosy was no longer seen in England from the fourteenth century. Pest Houses were typically away from the main thoroughfares, or on the periphery of villages, in order to achieve social distancing. Some of the houses had room to accommodate a surgeon or physician. They were not used exclusively for the plague, but were there to move people who *'frightened his neighbours'* [2]. It is surprising to note the range of payments made to those caring or overseeing the Pest Houses. The Pest Houses also gave an opportunity for some medical research to be undertaken, according to accounts [3]. The typical layout was the Pest House, with on one side Pest House meadow and on the other Pest House field. These Pestfields were sometimes used to increase capacity. Tents and temporary wooden buildings could be erected there to care for more sufferers. The tracks leading up to the houses were generally named either Pesthouse Lane or Close. Houses were best placed near water and lime; water to provide for those living in the Pest House and the lime to clean the houses with lime wash and use the lime when needed to hasten the decomposition of the dead. In general the Pest House is noted for having a very large and conspicuous chimney. It was believed that *'sweating to the utmost'* [4] would be the best method to eradicate the infection. The sick were kept in bed and they were sometimes tied to their beds. Broom was sometimes gathered and made into a beer to encourage sweating.

The houses described below are those that I have managed to find through ongoing research. It is of course by no means an exhaustive list, as every parish from 1665 had to allocate a house or shed for those with the plague.

There were five known Pest Houses in inner London about the time of 1665.

City Pest House – Bath Street. London EC1.
The Pest House was built in 1593 and could accommodate between 200 to 300 people. [5] From 1693 to 1718 it was used to care for sick French Protestant Huguenots, who fled from France, due to religious persecution. [6] A new French hospital *'La Providence'* replaced the original house from 1718, but was finally demolished in 1736. This Pest House was erected in 1630 by Sir. Theodore de Mayerne, physician to Charles I. [7] It was inspired and based on the *L'Hopital St Louis* in Paris. Sadly all that remains

of this largest Pest House in London is a plaque on the side of a multi-storey car park. This was the Pest House referred to as being in Bunhill Fields.

The Master of the City Pest House was Nathaniel Upton. He had the task of certifying the death of the inmates. The Pest House was demolished in 1736, but the site was later developed by the French Huguenots, who built their own French hospital here. Bath Street was originally known as Pest House Lane, but was renamed to avoid affecting the image of the Peerless Pool, used for swimming from the seventeenth century to 1869. [8]. In 1865 a new hospital was built in Victoria Park, Hackney and was later requisitioned to house the war injured in 1934. It then became used for sheltered housing for the elderly

Tothill Fields

The first known Pest House here was a shed for plague victims in 1638. A purpose built Pest House was built in 1651 at a cost of £250 by the philanthropist The lst Earl of Craven, a fellow of the Royal Society (1606-1697) and acquaintance of Pepys [9] He pioneered the further establishment of Pest Houses and gave money to assist the poor. The plague cottages consisted of a row of redbrick buildings. 'Five houses/ seven chimneys' and beside it was a plague pit. Pepys remarks in his diary

'how officers do bury the dead in open Tuttle fields' [10].

They were used as alms-houses in the early 1900's. This Westminster Pest House, was situated on marshy land between Millbank and Westminster Abbey. It was built on land known as The Sanctuary, behind Victoria Street. [11] . It is now known as Vincent Square. It is recorded that a woman called Barbara Spencer entered the Pest House late in her pregnancy and recovered, delivering a healthy baby six weeks into her stay. The Pest House could accommodate up to sixty people. [12]

Marylebone/Soho Pest House
The First Earl of Craven hired land in the Marshall Street area of Soho Fields and negotiated the development of a five acre site with William Lowndes of Chesham, Buckinghamshire. [12] The site was known as Clayfields. It served the parishes of St.Martin's, St. Clement's, St. Paul's Covent Garden and St. Mary Savoy. This area is now known as Golden Square. Dr.Tristan Inard was the physician and master of the Pest House. He was paid £170 per annum to care for the sick there. He also had another practice in Drury Lane, where he no doubt had seen many sufferers, as the 1665 outbreak started in that area. A large burial pit was situated nearby.

Mutton Fields, Marylebone
Another London site for a Pest House was a meadow in Marylebone known as Mutton Fields.

It was timber framed with a brick foundation [13]. The surgeon Dr Fisher was appointed there.

Stepney Pest House
The fifth Pest House in the outskirts of the City of London was situated in Stepney. The death toll here was particularly high, with at least 6,600 persons being carried away with the plague in 1665. Stepney, at the time, was a marshy area with pestilential air and the poor were huddled together in overcrowded conditions [14]

Further afield from Inner London were the following Pest Houses ….

Fulham Pest House, London
There was a Pest House on Hurlington Field. It was standing at the time of 1665, but was pulled down in 1681. It stood on ground where Hurlington Park is today [26]

Putney Pest House, London
A wooden Pest House comprising two rooms stood at the site of a row of almshouses near Putney Common and the Cricketers and The Spencer pubs along Lower Richmond Road, SW15. The brick Pest House was erected in 1665 but demolished in 1860, when it was no longer required. A vagrant was squatting there and it was felt that the place was so unhygienic that it was better to demolish it. [29] A white plague on the front of the cottages informs passers-by

of the former Pest House. Apparently 'twenty five persons died of plague in 1625 and seventy four in 1665, with only ten the following year' [30] A Pest House Charity was set up, which still awards grants to local organisations today.

Now, we will look outside London to Pest Houses sadly gone…..

Croxley Pest House, Hertfordshire
The Pest House was sited between Rickmansworth, Croxley and Loudwater, in South West Hertfordshire. It was situated by the side of a chalk stream River Chess. It had a distinct triple Tudor chimney, and was used from the seventeenth century to the mid nineteenth century. After it was used for plague victims it was divided into two tenements by John Morton in 1770 and rented out for £5 5 shillings a year. Joseph Weedon's family were installed to look after smallpox sufferers and they were paid five shillings weekly when they housed a smallpox victim. They were able to live there rent free. We can assume that they had contracted smallpox previously and were immune. The tithe map of 1839 shows the division of land between Pest House meadow and field. By 1834 the house and land was owned by the Watford Union and unfortunately it got into a state of disrepair over the years. After the Second World War the Dorrofield family came to make their home here.

The Dorrofield's were watercress growers and cultivated their crop in the River Chess. [15] In 1958 the house was demolished, but it is still possible to make out where the foundations were. An oil painting was completed by Tom Dorrofield, which is now stored at Three Rivers Museum, Rickmansworth.

A local family collected bricks from the derelict site and built a wall around their garden

Amersham Pest House, Buckinghamshire
Amersham in Buckinghamshire had a Pest House, although the records show that in 1665 there were only eleven deaths from the pestilence, in a population of approximately a 1000 [16]. It was built in 1625, half way up Gore Hill. It was a small two storey cottage, with walls covered in tar. There was a lime pit nearby in the dell. In 1906 the pest house was converted into a private dwelling called *'The Kennels.'* This house was demolished in 1964, when the road was widened. The position of the garden can still be seen by the garden plants that grow on the verge.

Beaconsfield Pest House, Buckinghamshire
Near to Amersham the town of Beaconsfield also had its allotted Pest House, about a mile north of the town. Fortunately they were spared the plague and the House was not used. [17]

Abbots Langley Pest House, approximate site The Royal Oak. Hertfordshire

Benskin Brewery deeds dated 1774 describe a building near here rated for use as a Parish Pest House. It was then altered to form a beer house between 1808 and 1827. It is thought that it was The Royal Oak. [18]

Watford Pest House, Hertfordshire.

The Watford Pest House was built at the end of Pest House Lane, which was renamed Willow Lane. The present hospital is located here too. The house was situated by the River Colne and near to lime kilns. After the plague, like so many of the Pest Houses, it remained in use for smallpox sufferers. [19] In 1754 it was noted that it was in a state of disrepair and unfit for the reception of the sick. However its condition must have been addressed as it is recorded that in 1758 a nurse was paid four pounds and ten shillings weekly to care for a smallpox patient. The governor at this time is recorded as William Jennings. In 1765 he was paid a salary of £70 per annum. A century later in 1893 a nurse was paid five shilling and five pence weekly, to care for those with smallpox. Surprisingly this wage was not a significant increase. It is listed as an isolation hospital by the following year of 1894 and leased to the Council in 1902. It was demolished in 1914

Chipperfield Pest House, Hertfordshire

This house served the parish of Chipperfield and Kings Langley. It was situated at the end of Pest House Lane, now renamed Croft Lane. There was a large pond near to the house. In 1838 the house was sold to John Parsley, Lord of the Manor. The 1839 tithe map clearly illustrates both Pest House field and Pest House meadow on either side of the house. [20]

Deddington Pest House, Oxford

This plague house/cottage was situated north of Deddington, off the Banbury Road and just before the turn to Milton. It was used for smallpox after the plague. It was still in use to care for smallpox victims in 1855, but was in ruins by 1896. There are references [21] to various disputes concerning the rental of the adjoining Pest House field, but eventually due to its dilapidated state the house was demolished in 1984. It does not appear to have been a substantial dwelling, as it's described as just a stone cottage or cow shed.

Redbourn, St Albans Pest House, Hertfordshire

The eighteenth century Parish Pest House was at Frogmore, on the south side of Redbourn Common. There was a row of cottages called The Wick. One of the cottages was run by Rebecca Brandreth as a Pest House until her death in 1799. [22]

St Albans, Park Street Pest House, St Stephens Parish, Hertfordshire

It stood on Hyde Lane, near a ford across the river. It was built in the fourteenth century to provide quarantine for the victims of the Black Death. It was used centuries later for isolation up to the mid eighteenth century. It was demolished sometime between 1872 and 1898 [23]

St Peter's Parish, St Albans, Hertfordshire

It is believed that there was a Pest House serving this parish along Sandpit Lane, now known as Oaklands Lane. It was closed in 1884. [24]

Sandridge Pest House, St. Albans, Hertfordshire

The Pest House stood on Park Croft, Hammond's Lane, Sandridge. It remained until at least 1776, but there is no trace now. [25]

Mount Pleasant, Stevenage Pest House, Hertfordshire

The Stevenage Pest Houses were a row of cottages. They were opened in 1765 to care for those with smallpox. When inoculation became common in 1799 the Pest Houses became redundant. By 1800 the cottages were let and eventually demolished. New housing stands on the site today.

Epping, Essex Pest House
Records [27] also list a Pest House on the north side of Lindsey Street, Epping. This was demolished by 1840. [28]

Ipswich Pest House – The Old Pest House, The Green, Hadleigh. IP7 6AE
This Pest House stood where Felixstowe railway runs behind Ascot Drive [31]. A Samuel Jacob was the master of the Pest House in 1665 and was paid thirty shillings weekly. Two or three nurses who worked there were paid five shillings a week each. Monies were provided from parish relief, but often towns had to contribute to the smaller parishes, who often fell into debt. Records show [32] that seventy five people were carried to the Pest House between April to November 1666, as the plague spread out from London. Sixty-five bodies were buried there and thirty-five people are said to have recovered and were sent home. The cold winter of 1666 brought an end to the plague.

Much Hadham Pest House, Hertfordshire
Bushwood Cottage, Bush Wood, Much Hadham. The boundary of the original house is still visible, although the building has gone. It is named as the Parish Pest House on the 1838 tithe map within Pest House Wood. Apparently it had the date 1767 over the doorway. After 1800 the cottage

became part of Lordship Farm and was used as a tied dwelling for farm labourers until 1914. It is still seen on the Ordinance Survey map of 1923. [33]

Cheshunt Pest House, Hertfordshire

Two tenements called the Pest Houses were founded in 1616 and stood in the south east corner of 13 Sandon Road. They were renovated in 1826 by George Robson to be used as parish almshouses. George Robson handed over the endowment to the Beaumont Trustees in 1859. They were demolished in the late twentieth century as a new arterial road was constructed nearby, with a new housing development [34]

Wigginton, Tring Pest House, Hertfordshire

The Pest House here was used until the 1870's. It was sited in North Pest House Wood, near the marlin chalk pits. It was the arrival of Lord Rothschild at Tring Park in 1872 which made the Pest House redundant, as he built a fever hospital in New Ground Road. The old Pest House then became a keeper's cottage. The local children are said to have gathered to see peacocks through the fence. [35]

Other known locations:

There are other known locations where Pest Houses once stood, but sadly have been lost to history.

Green Lane, Ardleigh, Colchester, Essex.

Dunstable Pest House, Bedfordshire stood on West Street at the junction of Drovers Way. It wasn't used after 1784.

Pest House Common, Queens Road, Richmond. Demolished in 1787.

Pest House, 7 Dukes Close, Farnham.

The Pest House, Bedlam Street, Hurstpierpoint Hassocks, West Sussex, BN6 9EW

Pest House Lane, High Cross, Ware, Hertfordshire. Plague sufferers were transported by the River Lea from London to be cared for in the country.

Pest House, Sevenoaks Common, Penshurst, Kent.

Pest House on Caddington Common, near Markyate, Hertfordshire. 1745

Maze Green Road, Bishop's Stortford, Hertfordshire. Formerly known as Pest House Lane. Pulled down in 1834.

The Pest House, on St Helen's, Isles of Scilly for sailors found to have plague –

It was never used. 1756 *'if plague shall appear on any ship, being northward of Cape Finisterre, the master shall proceed to St. Helen's pool.'*

(Hertfordshire data supplied with written permission from Hertfordshire County Council)

Chapter Eleven - Pest Houses still standing.

Again the list below of Pest Houses that are still standing is not exhaustive, but I hope it gives the reader a picture of the variety of houses that were used to isolate and care for the sick in the past. Historic England has complied a register of listed buildings and the following properties are listed there. [1]. I hope that those houses not yet registered will be recognised and recorded for posterity.

Hertford Pest House, Hertfordshire

The Old Pest House, Byde Street, Bengeo, Hertford is Grade 2 listed. It was built in 1763, principally for smallpox victims. Dr Thomas Dinsdale had the house built, and he was renowned for his work with smallpox. He devoted his life to smallpox prevention after seeing smallpox victims mixing in the streets, clearly suffering with unsightly scabs. He saw the urgency of isolation and containment, with 30 per cent mortality from the disease. Dinsdale lived in Port Hill House, which stood on the plot adjacent to the Pest House. It is thought that an earlier Pest House occupied this site. He also owned land nearby, for example in both Much and Little

Hadham. He was an MP for Hertford and was awarded the title Baron of the Russian Empire by Queen Catherine the Great after he inoculated her against smallpox. Inoculation was practised some time before vaccination became commonplace.

Cranbrook Pest House, Kent
The Pest House, Frythe Walk, Cranbrook, Tunbridge Wells, Kent is also Grade 2 listed. It is a two storey private dwelling, built originally in the sixteenth century. It still has the Pest House sign on the wall.

The Pest House at Godstone, Kent.
This Grade 2 listed house is situated at Bullbeggars Lane, Godstone, Tandridge Surrey. RH9 8BH. It is sited near water and was built in 1650.

Henley Pest House – Townlands Hospital, York Road, Henley-on-Thames, Oxfordshire.
(Grade 2 listed)
A workhouse was built in 1790 to accommodate 150 inmates and alongside this was erected a Pest House' which was used for the confinement of infectious cases. In 1794, the twenty-two year old poet Samuel Taylor Coleridge was an unwitting resident of the Pest House, having run away from Cambridge University where he had accumulated debts. Coleridge joined the Light Dragoons at Reading under the name of Silas Tomkyn Comberbache. When the Dragoons discovered

he was totally incapable of riding a horse, he was seconded to Henley and given the job of nursing a fellow recruit who had caught smallpox. The two men were confined in a small chamber for eight days and nights in foul conditions. Coleridge's time in the claustrophobic Pest House may have contributed to the imagery in the *Ancient Mariner*. [3]

'But oh! More horrible than that is the curse in a dead man's eye,

Seven days, seven nights, I saw that curse,

And yet I could not die' (The Ancient Mariner)

In 1948 with the advent of a National Health Service the new Townlands Hospital was developed on the site.

Grantham Pest House- White Cottage, 60 Manthorpe Road, Grantham, Lincolnshire. NG31 8DN. (Grade 2 Listed)

The original house was built in 1584, near to the River Witham [4] It was largely rebuilt in 1789 to contain the rising numbers of infectious patients. It was restored and extended in 1880, to be used as a private dwelling.

East Grinstead Pest House – Dorset Avenue, West Sussex. (Grade 2 Listed)

This is an attractive detached house built in the eighteenth century, principally for smallpox patients.

West Malling Pest House. Puckle Cottage, 91 Norman Road, West Malling, Tonbridge and Malling, Kent. (Grade 2 Listed.) [5]
Originally built in 1760 as a one up and one down house to isolate infected local residents. It is now an attractive three bedroomed property.

Potterspury Pest House – Pathfinder Cottage, Blackwell End, Potterspury, South Northamptonshire (Grade 2 Listed)**.**
Built in the seventeenth century to accommodate plague victims.

Southfleet Pest House – the house in the garden of Scadbury Manor, New Barn Road, Southfleet, Dartford, Kent. DA11 8EX (Grade 2 Listed).
This Pest House was built in the sixteenth century for travellers making a pilgrimage along Watling Street to Canterbury. The history of the area and Manor are fascinating, as the Walsingham family lived here during the Tudor period. Thomas Walsingham IV was knighted By Elizabeth I in 1597. The village sign illustrates this event. The Manor passed down to the Bessenden family and sadly burnt down in 1976. The Pest House building remains amongst the ruins of the Manor.

Guildford Pest House – The Old Cyder Cottage, 9 Pilgrims Way, Guildford, Surrey. (Grade 2 Listed)

This house was built in the sixteenth century as a two storey dwelling. It was known as The Old Cyder Cottage or Cyderhouse Cottage. It has been extended into a beautiful four bedroomed detached house. It is situated near the River Wey.

Linton Pest House – The Red Cottage, 12 Symonds Lane, Linton, South Cambridgeshire, Cambs. (Grade 2 Listed.)

The Red Cottage was built in 1748 to house any one with infectious diseases. The lane was initially named Union Lane instead of the usual Pest House Lane, but this was likely to be due to the Union Workhouse being sited just up the lane from the Pest House. It is now a private dwelling.

Wealden Pest House – Browndown Cottage, Cade Street, Heathfield and Waldron, Wealdon, East Sussex. (Grade 2 Listed.)

It is unclear whether this house was originally built in the sixteenth or seventeenth century. It is in a remote area and is now a private dwelling. An archaeological survey was undertaken in 2016, as the owner wished to lay a new concrete floor. Nothing of any historical interest was reported.

Fareham Pest House – Earl's Charity, 347 Hunts Pond Road, Titchfield Common, Fareham, Hampshire. (Grade 2 Listed).

As the road name suggests, there was a pond nearby. The house was built in the eighteenth century of red brick.

Maldon Pest House – 150-152 Fambridge Road, Maldon, Essex. (Grade 2 Listed)

It was built in the middle of the sixteenth century and converted now into a private dwelling. It was originally a timber framed two storey dwelling.

Hitchin Pest House - The New Found Out Public House, 181 Stevenage Road, Hitchin, Herts. (Grade 2 Listed).

This plague cottage was built at about 1612 and became an inn. The parish paid for a nurse to care for smallpox victims in the early eighteenth century. Records show that soap, gin, beer and playing cards were purchased, along with nutritious food. After smallpox inoculation the house was bought by John Marshall in 1818. It was named the 'New Found Out 'Inn. [6] A full history is referenced with kind permission of the current owners Jonathan and Emily Read. **[Appendix 3]**

Braughing Pest House – The Thatches, 39 Friars Road, Braughing, East Herts. (Grade 2 Listed.)

The present dwelling was built in the eighteenth

century. Prior to this there was another Pest House situated at Church End, Great Hormead. This was pulled down in 1895. Records show that a James Ginn and Elizabeth Howe lived here all their married life and cared for those afflicted with smallpox.

Charnwood Pest House – Pest Cottage, 26 School Lane, Woodhouse, Charnwood, Leicestershire. (Grade 2 Listed).
This cottage was built in the sixteenth century and was the home of writer Thomas Rawlins (1620-1670). He fled the plague from London in 1665 and was grateful to the villagers for their welcome. He left money in his will for the Rawlins School to be built in 1691.

The Pesthouse, Claygate Road, Maidstone, Kent. (Grade 2 Listed)
This timber framed red brick cottage was built in the sixteenth century, with added nineteenth and twentieth century facades.

The following houses still stand, but have not been awarded a listing, except the house at Northchurch (below).

Berkhamsted, Hertfordshire.
The area of Berkhamsted was a very unhealthy swampy area at the time of the Great Plague. There

are three houses still standing in Berkhamsted, Northchurch and Potten End. They are all private dwellings.

The Old Cottage, Shooters Way, Berkhamsted was originally a one up and one down home built in 1580, during the Elizabethan period. The present owner purchased it in 1982. The whole property needed renovation, as it had become uninhabitable. It was surrounded by a six acre farm and had a well at the end of the garden. There is a dewpond nearby.

Warren Cottage, New Road. Northchurch is sited well back from the road in Northchurch. This is the only house in Berkhamsted that is Grade 2 listed with Historic England. It was built in the seventeenth or eighteenth century and has been considerably extended since.

Moor Cottage,The Common, Potten End, Berkhamsted.
This was an eighteenth century parish Pest House, now in private hands and considerably enlarged. The house was built on The Common in 1774. Even in 1856 it was still being let, on condition that the tenants received smallpox sufferers.

Welwyn Pest House, Hertfordshire
A Pest House served the parish at Ninningswood Cottage, 2 Ninnings Lane, Welwyn, AL6 9TD.

It was used from the eighteenth century and from 1831 divided into three cottages for private purchase. One was pulled down and the two then joined into one.

Odiham Pest House, Hampshire
This Pest House was built between 1622 and 1625. It is tiny and measures only four metres by six metres. It has the trademark wide chimney and lies in a corner of All Saints churchyard. It was used until 1780 and then a purpose built Pest House housing smallpox patients was erected at nearby Colt Hill. The last resident died in 1930. Sadly by the 1970's it was in a poor state of decay and it was proposed that it be demolished. Fortunately a local Committee was formed, which worked to restore the house as a private museum. It was fully restored in 1981 and can be visited by appointment. [7]

Alton Pest House, Hampshire
Originally The Windmill at Alton was used, but Butts House, built in 1730 was the Star Inn and then the Butts Alehouse. It was used as the Pest House for smallpox patients in 1758. [8]

Findon Pest House, West Sussex.
This Pest House was extremely difficult to find. None of the local residents I asked had heard of it. Eventually I found it down a private track, about a mile north of the centre of Findon. There was

probably an older dwelling here originally in Saxon times and it could well have been used during the reign of Edward III, with the plague of 1348. Today the house is divided into two flint cottages. [9]

Hungerford Pest House, West Berkshire
There have been a number of dwellings used for housing plague victims. In 1848 a house was used for smallpox and is now divided into five units known as the Marshgate Apartments. [10] [11]

Woodstock, Oxford – Apple Tree Cottage
The Pest House in Woodstock was situated at the end of Pest House Lane. The road has since been renamed Rectory Lane. The house still stands and can be found at 23 Rectory Lane, Woodstock. It was used as a Pest House for smallpox victims from 1719 until 1765. [12]

Holmer Green, near High Wycombe, Buckinghamshire. Pear Tree Cottage, Pond Approach, Holmer Green. HP15 6SZ
Holmer Green was the first Pest House I visited. It is situated near a pond and a short distance away from the main village. It is a private dwelling and the owner believed it to have been used as a poor house/workhouse in 1704. The local history group also were unclear as to its purpose in the eighteenth century. The house has been extended and restored.

Chalgrave Pest House.- Hockcliffe Road, Chalgrave, Bedfordshire.
Hill Cottage was the parish Pest House, built in 1797 under instruction of the parish clerks. It is now a private dwelling and has been extended from the original two semi-detached cottages. Its use as a Pest House ended in 1837, when it was sold by the parish. A new Poor Law Workhouse was built at Woburn. [13]

Leighton Buzzard Pest House – The Anchor Beerhouse, Dunstable Road, Tilsworth, Bedfordshire. LU7 9PU
The Anchor was used as a Pest House between 1748 until 1823. It remains as a public house. It was used for smallpox victims mainly and was used between 1748 and 1823.

Framlington Pest House, Framlington, Suffolk
Built in the early seventeenth century. The sitting tenant would either stay to care for the infectious residents, or move elsewhere. Framlington Castle was also used as a Pest House. [14]

Ipswich Pest House/Isolation House, Ipswich, Suffolk
The house in Hadleigh now standing replaced the Pest House described previously.

West Meon, Petersfield, near Winchester, Hampshire

A Pest House was built in 1703 on "The Stroud'. This was an area of wasteland in Petersfield. It continued to be used to care for those with smallpox until 1834, when the Union Workhouse was built nearby in Love Lane. It has been renovated and enlarged and is now known as 'Mount Pleasant Farm.' [15]

Chapter Twelve - Isolation hospitals and fever nursing.

It became increasingly recognised that isolating the infected limited the chances that the infection would spread [1]. Quite a number of Pest Houses were used to care for smallpox sufferers and other infections, but many new isolation hospitals were built. As one disease receded another would increase and become more deadly, as with smallpox. The main factors that resulted in increased contagion was the influx of new immigrants, the mobility of populations, as travel increased, thirdly the impact of urbanisation.

Great advances were made in the nineteenth century in the understanding of diseases, treatments and diagnoses.

In 1676 the Dutch scientist Antonie van Leeuwenhoek identified bacteria, paving the way for the Italian Agostino Bassi to prove a silkworm disease was caused by a fungus in the early 1800's. [2] In 1864 Louis Pasteur (1822-96) laid out his germ theory of disease, which eventually became accepted. He demonstrated how germs fermented wine and soured milk. Pasteur was the inspiration for various followers. Joseph Lister developed antiseptics and Robert Koch (1843-1910) identified disease causing organisms;

anthrax in 1876, tubercle bacillus in 1882 and the following year cholera. [3] The distinctive nature of diphtheria was discovered in 1826, typhoid in 1837 and typhus in 1849. Prussian Rudolf Virchow, an eminent physician in the nineteenth century conceived the cell theory. He claimed that illnesses originated in individual cells. [4]

Gradually the terms fever hospital and isolation hospitals became synonymous and the terms will be used interchangeably here. Isolation hospitals were set up by local authorities, as was the case in earlier times with Pest Houses. This was in contrast to cottage hospitals and the large teaching hospitals which were privately funded by philanthropists, like Thomas Guy, who founded Guy's Hospital in London in 1721. The staff who worked in fever units were paid by the local authorities. The nurses would provide basic nursing care and importantly with diphtheria patients ensure a patent airway, if they needed tracheostomies. Healthcare was provided by the parishes up to 1834. Parish surgeons were only available to those receiving parish welfare.

Following the Public Health Acts of 1848 a Central Board of Health was established and in 1872 Medical Officers of Health (MOH) were appointed. Notification of infectious diseases became statutory in 1875, with the Public Health Act 1875. The Sanitary Act 1866 and the Public Health Act 1875 authorised local authorities to establish fever hospitals, but few complied before the 1890's. The Infectious Diseases Notification Act 1889 made it mandatory to notify disease in London and it became compulsory across England and Wales with the Extension Act of 1899. Prior to fever nurse training churches would fund parish nurses to help the sick in the community. It is interesting that still today there is a body of parish nurses across the UK funded by churches, although their role is supportive and pastoral, rather than statutory. [5]. After Queen Victoria's Golden Jubilee in 1887 special Queen's Nurses were appointed in her honour and their role included care of infectious patients. The Queen's Nurses Institute survives to this day, which awards the title Queen's Nurses to community nurses of distinction.

The first smallpox hospital in England was founded in 1746 at Cold Bath Fields, Clerkenwell in London. It was moved to a site at Highgate Hill in 1848, equipped with one hundred beds. It was a voluntary hospital and was fully used during the smallpox pandemic of 1870-1873

The Liverpool Fever Hospital was the first English hospital founded in 1801 to accommodate infectious patients other than smallpox. London had only two hospitals for infectious patients; the 100 bed Smallpox Hospital in Highgate and the London Fever Hospital with a capacity of 182 beds (1802), which was run on a voluntary basis. Institutions were established according to the local needs, for example Bedford had its own fever hospital in 1847.

Edward Jenner (1749-1823) initially experimented with the technique called variolation, or inoculation, in his quest to prevent death from smallpox. This was the deliberate infection of a person with a mild dose of the disease, by either scratching the skin using the exudate from smallpox sores, or inhalation through the nose.. This had long been practised in China, India, the Ottoman Empire and parts of Africa. Lady Mary Wortley Montagu introduced variolation to Western Europe from Turkey. Her three year old daughter was the first person to be inoculated in Western Europe. [6] The practice gained in popularity in the 1720's and Caroline, Princess of Wales, wife to the future King George II was persuaded to have her children inoculated against smallpox. Inoculation was risky, due to the risk of other infections, or dying from the disease. Fortunately, Jenner then went on to experiment with coxpox and developed vaccination against smallpox. The first Vaccination Act in 1840 enabled Poor Law Guardians to set up public vaccination services. [7] The Vaccination Act of 1853 made infant vaccination compulsory within the first three months. There was significant non-compliance and parents were coerced into having their children vaccinated, otherwise they could be fined or imprisoned. The medical profession believed that if vaccination was compulsory, especially for the vulnerable and high risk individuals like vagrants, that smallpox could be eliminated.

The Metropolitan Poor Act of 1867 legislated for the creation of the Metropolitan Asylums Board (MAB), which functioned as one hospital authority for the whole of London. The MAB had three functions – to establish hospitals for infectious diseases, care for the mentally ill and disabled and lastly to set up the first ambulance service. The MAB set up nine acute fever hospitals and one temporary one. The MAB introduced radical changes. It set up the land ambulance service in 1881 and the river service in 1884. [8] In 1871 the Local Government Board replaced the Poor Law Board in England and Wales. However local authorities were reluctant to set up their own isolation hospitals, favouring instead the use of offshore ships as floating hospitals, using the new river system. Checks at the port entries were important to ensure that travellers to the country were not transmitting infections, which has been a focus of recent efforts with CoV Sars 2. Port Sanitary Authorities (PSA's) were introduced in 1872, called the 'English system' [9]. Ships with visible signs of disease were disinfected and the infected passengers transferred to isolation hospitals. The rest of the crew and passengers were quarantined. The quarantine hulk *Dreadnought* moored at Greenwich took in smallpox victims during the epidemic of 1871-72. Other MAB ships were the *Atlas, Endymion and Castalia,* moored in the Thames estuary. The restrictions at ports were hugely unpopular, due to the impact on trade, but was seen as necessary to avoid spread of infection into the country. Quarantine was finally abolished in 1896, when infectious diseases had become less prevalent and containable in medical institutions.

The epidemics of 1881 and 1884 confirmed that smallpox spread from hospitals [10]. Therefore in 1882 Dr Thorne wrote a Report on the use of hospitals for infectious diseases and his key recommendations included a more proactive approach to the management of infections. He said that specialist hospitals should be built in advance for future epidemics, rather than attempt to accommodate infected people in hospital units not fit for purpose.

Viruses were only initially discovered in the 1890's. The Isolation Hospitals Act of 1893 gave authority to County Councils to require local authorities to build isolation hospitals. Three years after this Act an isolation hospital was opened in Tolpits Lane, Watford and continued in use until 1982. [11] The size and quality of these hospitals varied across the country. The larger units in urban areas found it easier to attract staff.

No and type of institution	No of beds	Average no of beds
755 fever hospitals	31,149	41
700 Poor Law Infirmaries	94,001	134
594 General Hospitals	31,329	53
363 Smallpox hospitals	7,972	22
222 Special Hospitals	13,654	62

Source: *Forty-fourth Annual Report of the Local Government Board, 1914-1915. Part 111.-a).*
Public Health and Local Administration. London. HMSO. 1916. Cd 8197, pp26-27

As you can see from the above table, fever hospitals were the most common type of institution at the outbreak of the First World War. By 1922 every district had its own isolation or fever hospital, caring for those with conditions such as smallpox, cholera, measles, diphtheria, typhus, scarlet fever and whooping cough (pertussis).

History is marked by the achievements of key female reformers. Elizabeth Fry (1780-1845) was the Quaker prison reformer, Louisa Twining (1820-1912) campaigned for trained nurses to care for the workhouse sick in separate infirmaries, and Octavia Hill (1838-1912), worked in the slums of London. Florence Nightingale (1820-1910) met opposition from her family when she committed herself to caring for the sick and nursing during the Crimea. Florence believed in the miasmic theory, stating:

'the first canon of nursing....to keep the air he breathes as pure as the external air.' [12].

Staffing these fever and smallpox hospitals was a real challenge, partly due to the risks of contagion, but also due to the lack of opportunities to progress in general nursing. A Watford resident lamented the lack of a Resident Medical Officer at the Watford Isolation Hospital [13] and the lack of trained nurses. Records from the London Smallpox Hospital in Highgate highlight the fact that medical staff contracted the disease, as has been the case with coronavirus.

Beatrice Hopkinson [14] became a fever nurse in 1913, rather than a general nurse, probably because of limited finances. The fever nurse training was a much shorter course and often subsidised. The teaching hospitals often required fee payments to enter nurse training. Fever nurse training was often inadequate and not standardised. Dr. Alec Gordon, writing in the *British Journal of Nursing* in January 1907 *'The Position of the Isolation Hospital in the training of the Nurse'* [15] said that training in a number of hospitals was below standard.

It took some time for fever nurses to achieve registration on the Nurses Supplementary Register. Doctors were the first health professionals to achieve registration under the Medical Act 1858, followed by midwives in 1902, after a number of years struggling to do so. The Fever Nurses Association (FNA) was established in 1908. Its aim was to maintain a standard of training and keep a register of trained fever nurses.

The FNA syllabus was approved in MAB fever hospitals in July 1909. Training took two years, with an optional extra two years to achieve state registration. Similarly State Registered Nurses could undertake fever nursing if they completed an extra year's training. The training was rigorous and included the instruction on performing a tracheotomy in emergency situations, when dealing with cases of diphtheria. In 1909 there were over 700 fever hospitals in the country, employing about 15,000 nurses [16].

The College of Nursing was established in London in 1916, followed by the Nurses Registration (England and Wales) Act 1919. There were five supplementary parts, fever nursing being one of them. It was never seen as prestigious as entering the main register and yet these nurses were caring in life and death situations.

Gradually diagnostic tests were developed to identify infections. The Dick and Schick tests were carried out to test for scarlet fever and diphtheria. Antitoxins were available when needed in the late nineteenth century and resulted in a marked drop in case fatalities. An Englishman W.M. Stanley identified a flu virus first and an American Salk in 1933 perfected the first anti-viral vaccine [17]

With the outbreak of the First World War, fever hospitals were filled with sick soldiers. Tetanus was a particular problem in the trenches. [18] Soldiers who were being cared for in private homes and camps were protected from community contagion by red crosses being painted on the doors [19], a practice previously described, which was adopted hundreds of years earlier. The dreaded fever cart was used to transport infected persons at night in a similar fashion to the pest coaches of the 1600's. The MAB horse drawn ambulances were last drawn on 14 September 1912 and the MAB finally closed in 1930.

The last smallpox epidemic in Britain was 1901 -1902. Its final eradication, as declared by the World Health Organisation (WHO), occurred in 1980; the last known case reported in Somalia in 1977. Specialist hospitals were set aside replacing the Pest Houses. Smallpox was caused by a small virus, spread mainly by droplets. There was a ten to twelve day incubation period. Symptoms would suddenly develop, including high temperature, muscular pains, nausea and vomiting and then the typical rash. The rash started out as macules, which then became pustular. No one was immune, as Queen Elizabeth I nearly died from it, but Mary II did in 1694 and King Louis XV in 1774. [20]. Smallpox nurses were required to keep to a strict regime of quarantine. They wore hooded linen overalls called 'wrappers' and overshoes [21]. Although it is officially eradicated there is still no proven antiviral agent to treat smallpox. Supportive care and antibiotics for any secondary infection are all that is available in our armoury.

By 1914 there was a real division regarding the enforcement of enteric inoculation. Some argued that compulsory inoculation interfered with human rights, whilst the pro inoculation lobby, like the medical practitioner Sir William Osler stated 'the microbe kills more than the bullet.' [22]

In 1929 the work undertaken by Boards of Guardians transferred to the London County Council (LCC). The MAB was wound up, with poor law institutions evolving into general hospitals.

The advent of the National Health Service (NHS) in 1948 resulted in significant organisational changes for the hospitals. Fever and smallpox hospitals transferred to the management of Regional Hospital Boards. These were great losses to local authorities, but it was becoming clear that as infections were better controlled and treated that it seemed better to accommodate patients near to diagnostic services in general hospitals. The spur to vaccination was smallpox. Those who developed immunity to smallpox were asked to nurse the sick with smallpox. Some of the smallpox and fever hospitals were retained for specialist care and others used for geriatric, mental illness and physical disability services.

Nutrition had improved, immunisations and antibiotics were available and fever nurse training gradually came to an end. The antibiotic streptomycin became available in the early 1950's and penicillin in the 1940's. The bacterium staphylococcus aureus was first identified in England in 1961 [23] soon after methicillin was introduced. The Fever Register for England and

Wales was finally closed on 31 December 1967.

The wisdom of closing the fever hospitals and stopping the fever nurse training can now be questioned, with the recent pandemics we have endured. We could have minimised hospital acquired infections today by avoiding admissions to general hospitals and using isolation institutions instead. The needs of society can change, as we have witnessed at the start of 2020.

Vaccination has enabled us to eradicate and control infections. Today plague is not worth vaccinating against as although it still exists, there are few cases [24].

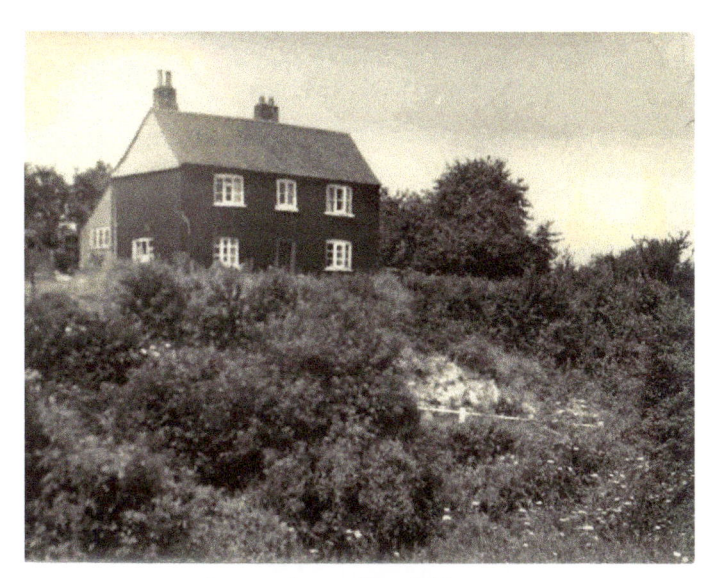

Amersham Pest House
Amersham Museum

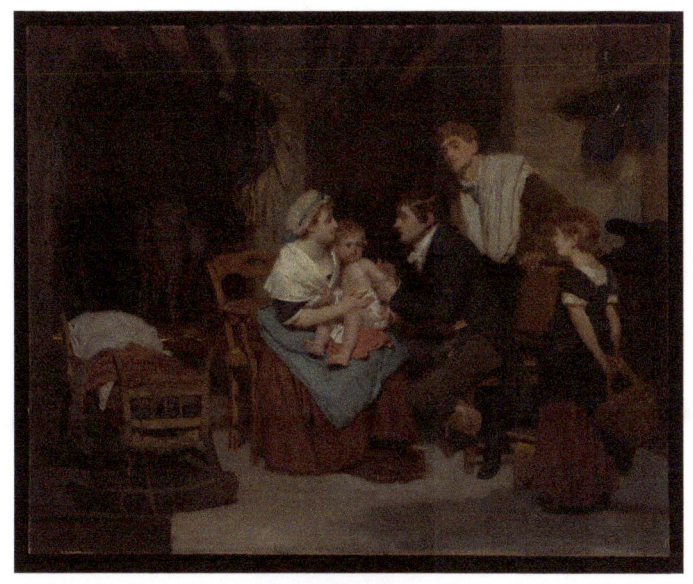

vaccination
Look and Learn

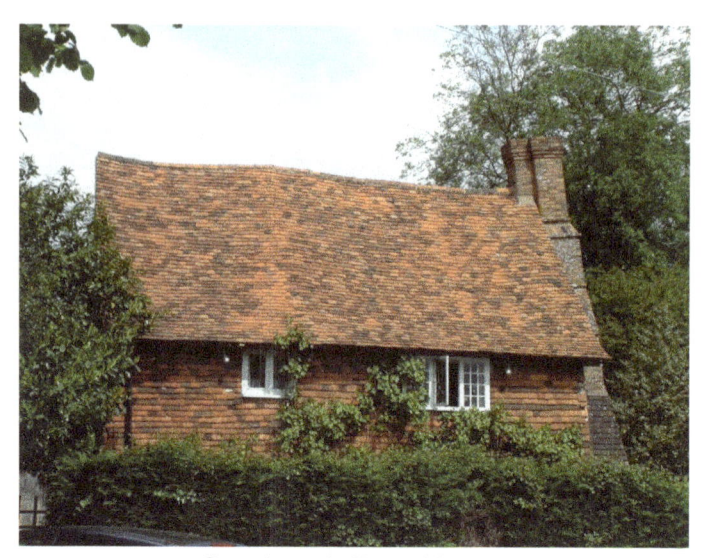

Cranbrook Pest House
Author

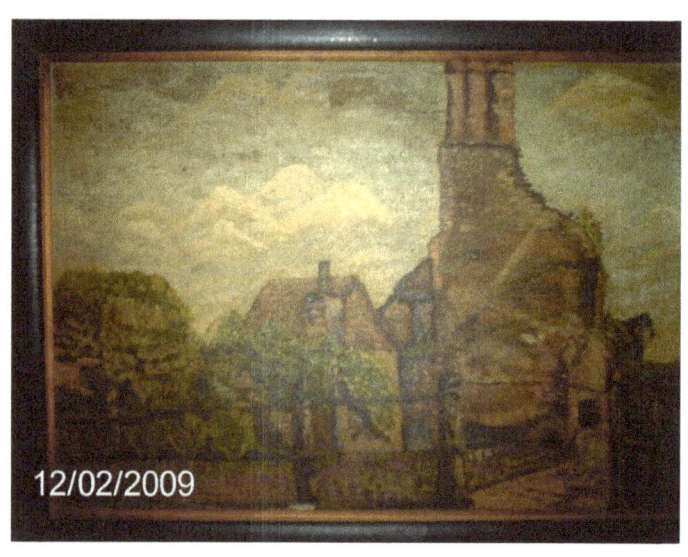

Croxley Pest House
Author

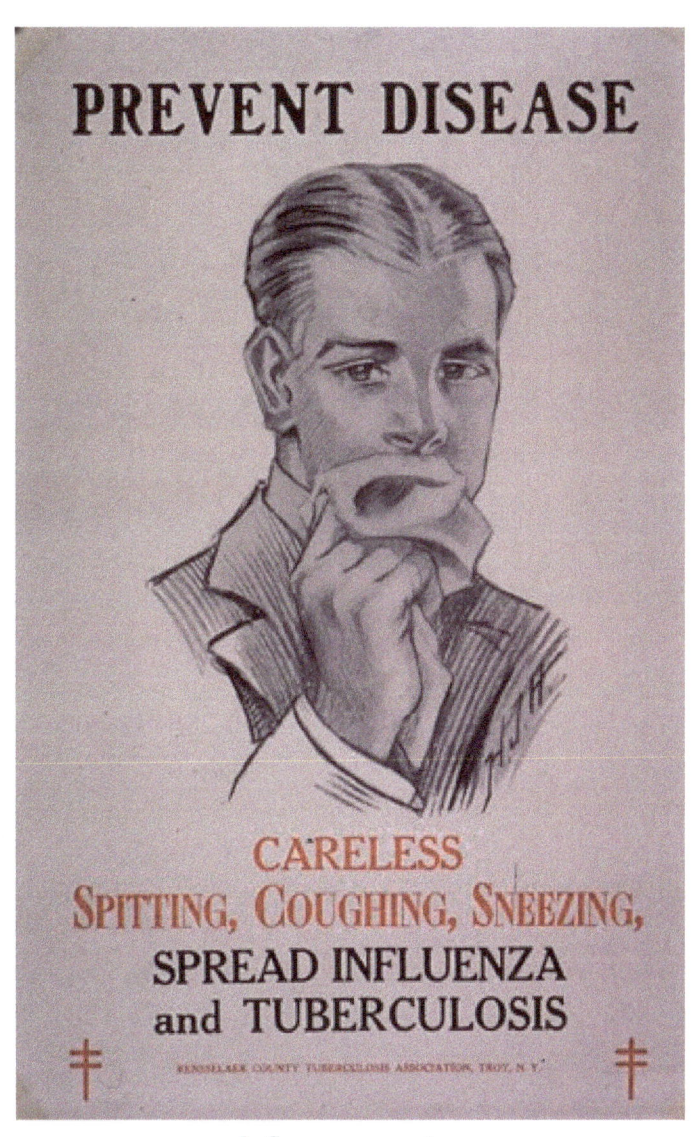

Influenza poster
Look and Learn

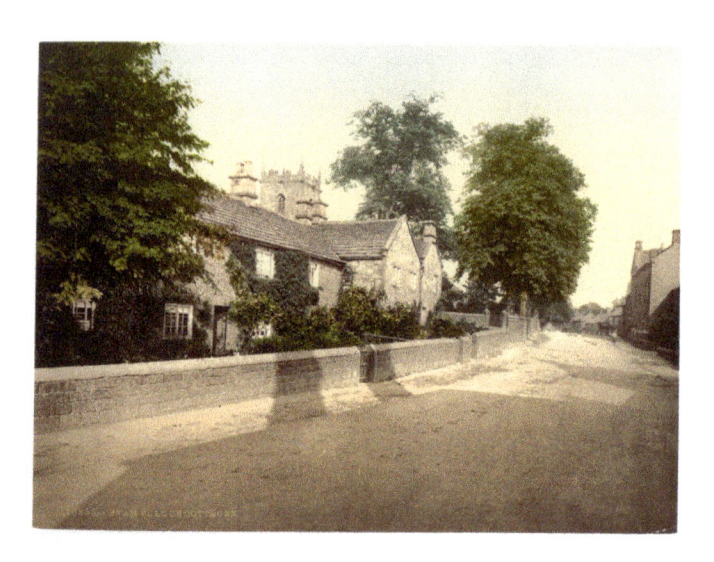

Eyam plague cottages
Look and Learn

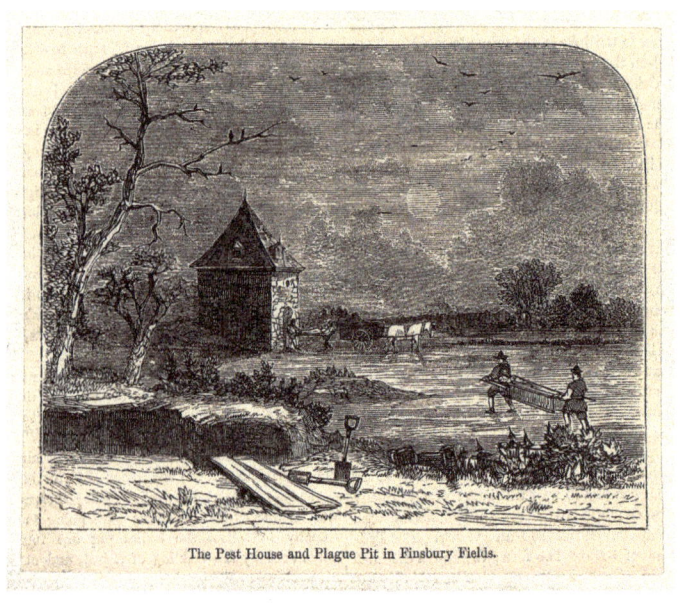

The Pest House and Plague Pit in Finsbury Fields.

Finsbury fields pest house
Look and Learn

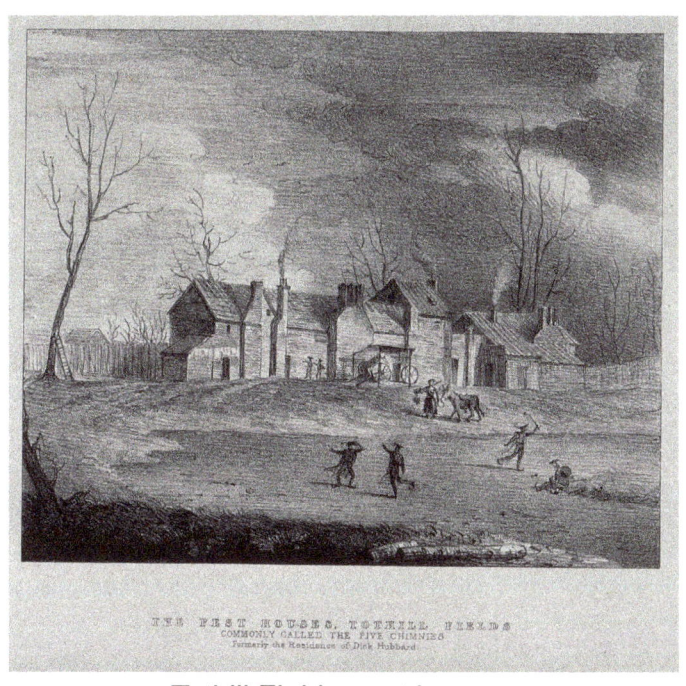

Tothill Fields pest houses
Look and Learn

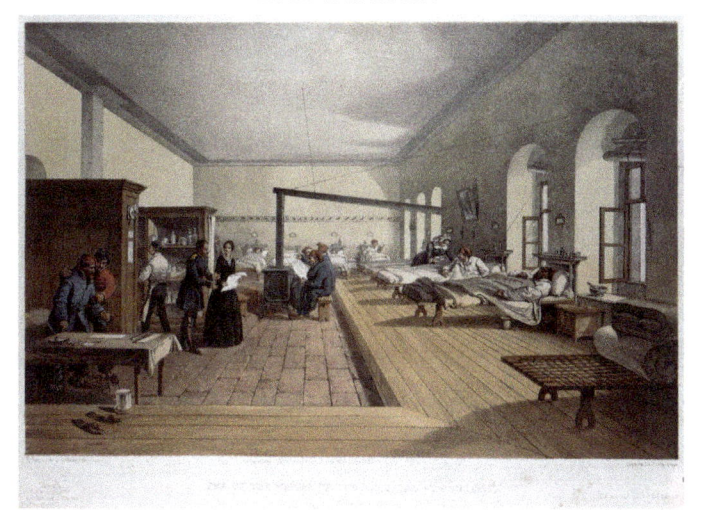

Florence Nightingale ward
Wellcome Collection

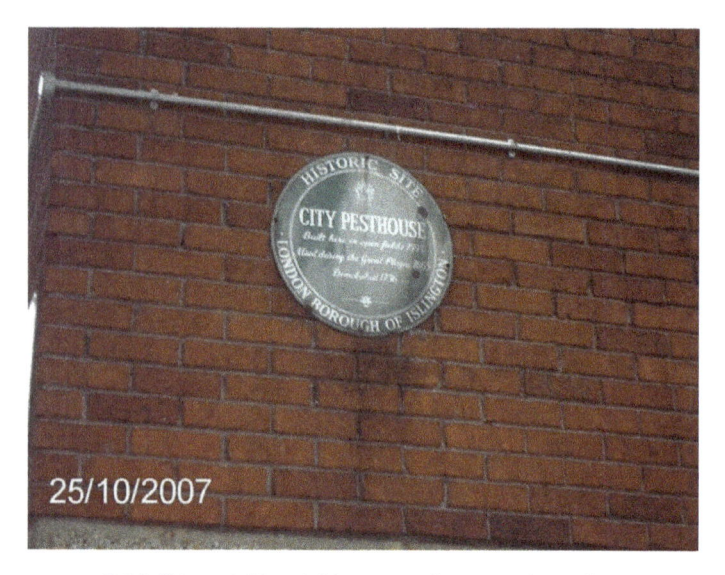

Old Street Pest House plaque, London
Author

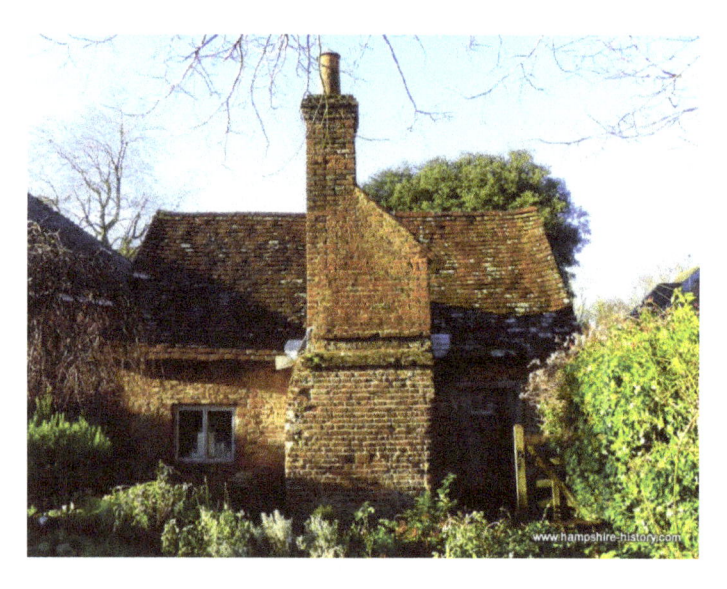

Odiham Pest House, Hampshire
Author

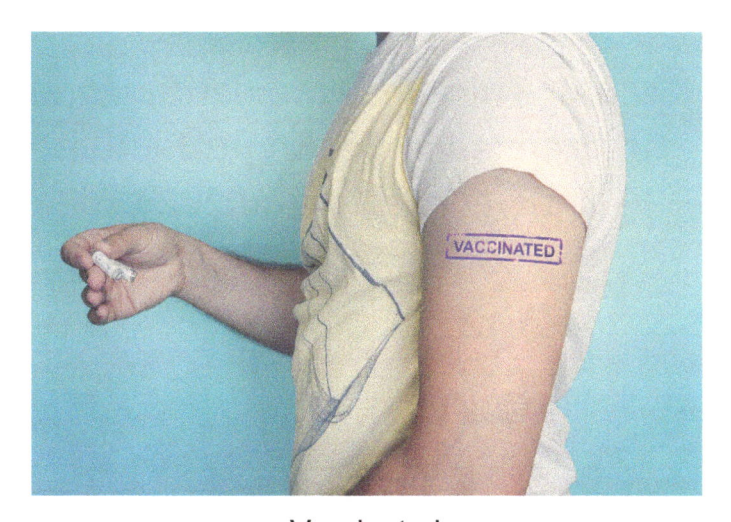

Vaccinated
Shutterstock

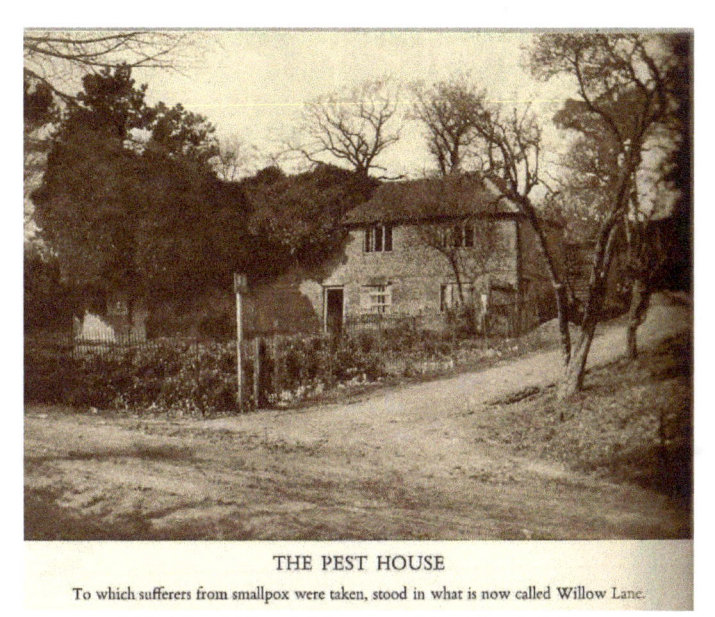

THE PEST HOUSE
To which sufferers from smallpox were taken, stood in what is now called Willow Lane.

Watford Pest House, Hertfordshire
Watford Museum

Chapter Thirteen - Similarities and Differences in health protection between 1665 and 2020

Similarities between the plague (1665) and coronavirus (2020) :

1665	2020
• FEAR! Lack of understanding. • Zoonotic transfer – animal to human • Deprivation risks • Crowds and lack of space. • Bills of Mortality • Social control – watchmen/rods and crosses/travel • Charles ll/ Parish relief • Pest Houses • Economic impact of public health measures	• Fear- lack of understanding • Zoonotic transfer – animal to human • Deprivation risks • Crowds and space • Registering and epidemiology • Social distancing/ closure/masks/travel • Central/local gvt support. Furlough schemes. • Nightingale hospitals • Economic impact of public health measures.

As described in 1665 people were really fearful, as they had no real comprehension of the spread of disease. They believed they had incurred God's wrath and had to pay retribution for their sins. They looked to the stars and comets or simple quackery. Physicians and philosophers devised their own theories as to cause and effect. Today coronavirus has taken the world by surprise and although it was understood that it was a SARs virus belonging to the cold virus family, there was initially little understanding regarding its infectivity or virulence. To achieve approval for vaccines so quickly is simply incredible and we should be proud of our vaccine record in the UK.

It soon became apparent who the high risk groups were today, as they were in the seventeenth century. Disease hits the poor hardest, who generally live in overcrowded, poor conditions. Those with chronic conditions have been the most vulnerable.

Records were kept during the Great Plague in each parish and weekly Bills of Mortality were published. These Bills go back to 1562, as the wealthy wished to have sufficient warning of an impending wave of the plague or pox.

Hearth tax was introduced in the 1660's [1] also illustrated the epidemiology of the diseases and confirmed that those wealthier inhabitants with hearths to pay for, often escaped the plague. Today a vast amount of epidemiological data is available. [2] The media bombarded us daily with the latest incidence, prevalence, morbidity and mortality statistics, but as in 1665 the statistics can be manipulated to give a certain impression about the extent and trends of a disease.

Social distancing was practiced in the past, as it has from 2020. People during the plague years were ordered to carry rods of various colours and length to alert the parish that they were infected or belonged to an infected house. We employed social distancing, adopting a two metre rule, wearing masks and in relevant situations full personal protective equipment. (PPE) [3] Masks are still required in some settings and institutions, in particular travel to certain destinations. Proof of vaccination is also requested in a few areas.

Parishes collected parish relief to support those who suffered from plague and other illnesses leading to incapacitation. The present Government spent a huge amount on furlough schemes, [4] support grants and money for track and trace and equipment. Inevitably, as in 1665, there is a trade-off between measures to contain contagion and measures to protect the economy.

The Nightingale hospitals were built at great speed and at great expense to accommodate the projected thousands of anticipated patients. In 1665 Charles II decreed that every parish must allocate a tent, hut or house to serve as a plague house. They were used throughout the Great Plague, so there the similarities between the past and today diverge. We can now look at the differences between the two periods in the way that the plague and coronavirus have been managed and consider lessons learnt.

Differences between the plague (1665) and coronavirus (2020):

1665	2020
- Social media - Ethnic differences - Bacteria v. virus - Gender differences - Age – indiscriminate - Lifestyle risks - Cats and dogs – slaughtered - No contact tracing - Charles ll looked at past events - Hospitals were not used	- Technology/ global spread - Black and Asian x 4 likely to die. - Antibiotics ineffective - Females /males - Age – increased risk with elderly - Lifestyle – obesity/ smoking - Pet ownership increased - Track and trace - Following the science - Hospital acquired infection

The world is a very different place today, compared to life in Stuart England. There was no social media, except the handwritten notes and Bills. Technology has changed all that and news, including fake news travels fast. We live in a world of mistrust and conspiracy theorists. Although communication was so different there seems to have been some misreporting of diagnoses of the plague. People understandably would wish to hide contagion in their household and there are records of searchers being bribed, in order to not disclose outbreaks of infection.

There were no ethnic differences to the risk of plague, in stark contrast to the greatly increased susceptibility to coronavirus if you are Asian or of African origin. [5] It seems to be because of genetic differences, but may also be linked to darker skinned people being more prone to vitamin D deficiency.

Yersinia pestis is a bacterium and responds to antibiotics, whereas coronavirus or Co Sars 2 is a virus. Viruses behave differently and mutate endlessly, particularly if transmitted via immunocompromised individuals. Men and women died and suffered the plague in equal measure, although more women died as they seemed to be the ones caring for the sick and being employed as nurses and searchers. Men are more at risk of coronavirus, due to hormonal differences. The male hormone testosterone and the number of ACE 2 receptors [6] that line the respiratory tract in men provide attachment points for the virus to embed and multiply. Women also have the same cells, but in much smaller amounts.

As well as gender differences, there are age differences between the two diseases. Young and old were dying of the plague, whereas very few young people have had significant symptoms from covid and most have been asymptomatic.

Lifestyle factors appear to be linked to risk factors. Sedentary lifestyles and being overweight are linked to greater vulnerability to covid 19.

Although the 'track and trace' system

experienced challenges, the Local Government Association (LGA) applauded the success of local contact tracing [7]. If the national online team were unsuccessful in making contact, then the case was transferred to local environmental health teams in Councils. Data for the week ending 14 October 2020 showed that 94.8 per cent of people were located and instructed to self-isolate, compared to only 57.6 per cent reached through the National Call Centres. [8].

Charles II sought assistance from the scientists and looked back at previous periods of plague to consider the best way forward. Pest Houses had been used in an ad hoc fashion, but Charles II decided a consistent, co-ordinated, joined up approach was needed.

As I will discuss in the last chapter I believe the use of the general hospitals today has been a significant mistake in the management of the most recent pandemic and led to the spreading of covid infection.

Chapter fourteen - Reflections

Although there were warnings that a pandemic was imminent, the world seems to have been taken by surprise when coronavirus spread so rapidly in 2020. As we have seen in the seventeenth century, plague outbreaks were regular and expected.

A real threat facing mankind is the rise of zoonotic diseases and bioterrorism. [1] These are diseases that jump from animals to human and then spread. They are increasing because we are changing our relationship with farmed and wild animals. They are linked to deforestation, the encroachment into previously uninhabited areas and the hunting and sale of animals in markets.

'The more we change nature, the more likely we are to see diseases like Covid-19 emerging'

says Kate Jones, Professor of Ecology at University College, London. We could face a far worse pandemic in the future and need to learn the lessons from Covid-19. [2]

An important lesson we can learn from the time of the Great Plague is the importance of isolation of the infected from healthy communities. Plague cottages and tents were rapidly erected, designed to remove those who posed a risk to the health and wellbeing of others. It was understood that the general hospitals like St Bartholomew's should not accept plague sufferers, as the contagion would rampage through the institution. The Health Service Journal (HSJ) has published their analysis into hospital acquired covid infection. Data indicates almost 25 to 40 per cent of coronavirus has been contracted in hospitals [3]

Unfortunately our isolation units in the UK have mostly been demolished and are unavailable. Nightingale hospitals were built rapidly, but the appropriate staff to man them was not available.

Messaging in the seventeenth century remained consistent with simple instructions and penalties. As infection rates have soared today the messages have changed, making it difficult to achieve compliance and trust. Heavy handedness also seems not to be the best policy, if we are to see whole communities working together to control and eventually beat the virus.

However we need to also look at the things that have worked well. We should applaud the incredible speed of vaccine research and manufacture. The vaccine rollout has been exemplary and enabled us to look ahead to regaining a sense of normality again. [4] Charles Dickens wrote about the delays during the diphtheria crisis in 1856 (known as the 'Boulogne fever' at the time, as it seemed to originate there). [5] The scientific name was conceived by Pierre Bretonneau. Diphtheria caused the development of a leathery membrane covering the larynx, which when severe required a tracheostomy. By 1860 diphtheria was better understood, but it wasn't until the 1920's that a vaccine was developed and the vaccine given free to children in the 1940's.

Similarly a tetanus vaccine was developed in the 1920's, but wasn't extensively used until the Second World War [6]

In the seventeenth century a parish relief levy was introduced to support the parishes during the plague. The local parish could call upon the Government for extra assistance when required. We saw the same today with the furlough scheme and local support schemes, both statutory and voluntary. We have seen communities work together and support their neighbours.

Plagues and pandemics have impacted societies; both economically and politically. The Black Death of 1348, for example, overturned feudal hegemony. This recent pandemic has transformed society in various ways, but it is too soon to say with any certainty how it has changed society in detailed terms.

As in the past fake news travels fast, so in response the World Health Organisation set up a web page to address common myths about the disease [7]

We face a range of pandemics; we must not forget the chronic pandemic that has been highlighted throughout recent times –

'non-Communicable' diseases – cardiovascular disease, diabetes, cancer, and mental health – are the pandemics of the twenty-first century [8]

So there we have it – I take my hat off to Charles II, and his wisdom at the time of the Great Plague of 1665. Dr.Thorne in 1882 was also a real visionary, who called for a proactive approach, and pandemic preparedness. The setting up of parish plague cottages showed compassion, foresight and a real understanding of what public health in action really meant.

APPENDIX 1

Shakespeare's plays that allude to the plague.

William Shakespeare was born in Stratford in April 1564. The plague swept across the country in waves during his life, notably in 1564, 1582 and 1592-4 and was the most unrelenting over the period 1603 to 1610, during the reign of James I. Over this period of seven years the theatres were mostly kept shut and the plays Shakespeare wrote over this time reflect the mood of the country. He used the term plague metaphorically in some plays as an expression of rage and passion. Over this time Shakespeare's plays were performed at the King's Court. The people at this time learnt to live with the ravages of plague, never knowing when a lull in infection would turn again. Shakespeare's life is undocumented over the lost years of 1585 to 1592, when there was a relative period of calm from the pestilence. It may be that at this time he travelled the world. Tragically his son Hamnet died in 1597. We do not know if he actually died of the plague or not. No one dies of the plague in any of the plays, despite references to the infection.

The birth of his granddaughter Elizabeth in 1608 may have helped Shakespeare change his view on life and adopt a more optimistic outlook.

The only play where he describes how the plague directly affected the outcome of the play is-

Romeo and Juliet. (probable date 1594)
This romantic tragedy is set in Verona. Friar Lawrence was delayed in sending a message because "searchers of the town ... sealed up the doors and would not let us forth." Mercutio when speaking of the two families the Capulets and Montagues says "a plague on both your houses." Other plays that refer to the plague include-

Love Labour's Lost (probable date 1595)
Another Elizabethan comedy set in Navarre. Berowne speaks of the passion between the main characters –"deceive me not now, Navarre is infected" and later in the play
"it is a plague that Cupid will impose". "a fever in your blood! Why, then incision…"
"Light wenches may prove plagues to men forsworn"
"Thus pour the stars down plagues for perjury" laments Berowne, as he interjects between Ferdinand and Rosaline.
"I am sick I shall leave it by degrees….write Lord have mercy on us … They have the plague and caught if of your eyes! These Lords are visited, you are not free; for the Lord's tokens on you do I see."

Much Ado About Nothing (probable date 1598)
Beatrice and Benedick are the principal characters in this comedy. Speaking of love Beatrice states "he will hang upon him like a disease: he is sooner caught than the pestilence".

Twelfth Night (probable date 1601)
A popular comedy, mixing mournful sorrow and cheeky humour. Olivia reflects on the fact that "ever so quickly may one catch the plague." Referring to a passion of love and lust.

Hamlet (probable date 1601)
Set in Denmark, this play is arguably the greatest tragedy in the English language.
"this now the very witching time of night, when churchyards yawn, and hell itself breathes out, contagion to this world."

King Lear (probable date 1605)
This is a play about the bases of human nature and man's dignity.
King Lear curses his daughter Goneril. "Thou art a boil, a plague sore" At the end of the play King Lear cries "a plague upon you, murderers, traitors all."

Macbeth (probable date 1605)
Shakespeare may well have been drawing on the plot to kill King James I in the Gunpowder Plot of that same year. "Sighs and groans ..... dying when they sicken"

Timon of Athens (probable date 1607).
Timon is an Athenian noble who berates humanity and is filled with self-pity. Timon says to a passing visitor – "Be as a planetary plague, when Jove will o'er some high-viced City hang his poison, in the sick air."

Coriolanus (probable date 1607)
This play is a political play that in essence dissects democracy and compares it to autocracy or dictatorship. Coriolanus spits at the plebeians "you herd of boils and plagues… all the contagion of the south light on you, you shames of Rome."

A Winters Tale (probable date 1610).
We see from here on a gradual lifting of mood in Shakespeare, as the end of the seven year period of plague comes to a close.
This play has the same theme running through it as King Lear, as Shakespeare centres it on the father daughter relationship, but he retells this play to have a happy ending. Leontes, King of

Sicily says "the blessed Gods, purge all infection from our air."

The Tempest (probable date 1611)
Another romance and the last play attributed solely to Shakespeare. Prospero cries "poor worm thou art infected, this visitation shows it" when Ferdinand falls in love with Miranda.
(Dunton-Downer, L & Riding, A. *Essential Shakespeare Handbook.* London. Dorling Kindersley. 2004)

APPENDIX 2:

The Diary of Samuel Pepys. Edited by R.C.Latham & W.Matthews. Vol.V1. 1665

Quotes regarding the plague of 1665 in Pepys diary:

- Great fears of the Sickenesse here in the City, it being said that two or three houses are already shut up. [30 April p.93]

- All the news is of the Dutch being gone out..... and of the plague growing upon us in this town and of remedies against it; some saying one thing, some another. [24 May. p.108]

- This day.... I did in Drury-Lane see two or three houses marked with a red cross upon the doors, and "Lord Have Mercy upon us " writ there.... So that I was forced to buy some roll tobacco smell and chaw....[7 June. p.120]

- The plague is come into the City (though it hath these three or four weeks since its beginning been wholly out of the City) but where should it begin but in my good friend and neighbour's,

Dr.Burnett in Fanchurch-street...[9 June p.124]

- Saw poor Dr.Burnett's door shut ... he hath gained great goodwill among his neighbours; for he discovered it himself first, and caused himself to be shut up of his own accord....[11 June p.125]

APPENDIX 3:

History and development of the Hitchin Pest House.

"The Well", 181 Stevenage Road, Hitchin, Hertfordshire
Design & Access Statement
May 2010

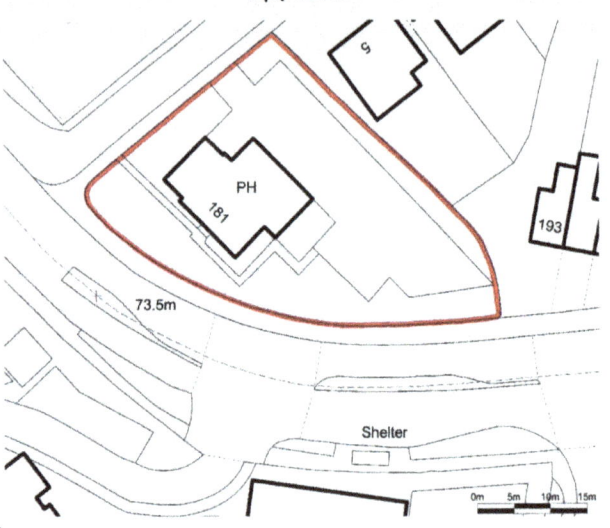

Introduction

1. "The Well" (known as "The New Found Out" Public House when Listed) is Listed Grade II, the list description being:-

    "Said to have been formerly the Pest House. C17-C18 origin, red brick gabled north wing, modern south wing. The north wing is of 2 storeys and attics with diagonal brick gables, band below and carried over the upper storey window of the side elevations; tiled roofs with gabled dormer on south east side. South gabled front has partly blocked original window in gable, large upper storey window opening with cambered head, partly filled in, band, window opening on ground floor. The north west side has 2 very large blocked upper storey windows"

2. The building is not located within a Conservation Area. The area is zoned for residential development.

3. The history of the building is set out below. There have been many attempts to run it as a Public House, but all have ended in failure. It has now been closed and sold off by Punch Inns.

"The Well", 181 Stevenage Road, Hitchin, Hertfordshire
Design & Access Statement

History

4. The building is thought to date from the early 17th century, probably originally a dwelling. Towards the mid 1700's it was leased to Hitchin Parish Vestry as an isolation unit for people suffering from contagious illnesses such as the plague or small pox, it was then known as the 'The Pest House'. In 1818 the building was owned by John Marshall of Hitchin, brewer, and occupied by Edward Ball, though apparently not as an inn. It wasn't until 1909 when it was bought by Simpsons Brewery who first opened it as a pub with the name 'The New Found Out'. This name was chosen because the landlord at the time had come from the (Old) Found Out and brought the name with him. Sometime in the 1950's the pub was taken over by Greene King and continued to trade until it was closed in 1969. For the next 10 years the premises were unoccupied and the building started to deteriorate into a serious state of dilapidation. The building was Listed in the 1970s. In 1976 Greene King made application to demolish the building, which was refused. In 1977 the pub, still closed, was sold to a Mr. Simpson of Pirton. In October 1978 the pub was sold again and opened as a restaurant. This endeavour started off successfully but after a year or so the 'New Found Out' reverted back to being a traditional public house. In 1986 it was owned by Messer's Fuller, Smith & Turner of Chiswick, then for the next few years it was bought and sold by several breweries and other companies until ending up in the ownership of Inn Business Limited. In May 1997 the property was leased to Terence Reeder who was responsible for renaming the Public House to 'The Wishing Well', a controversial move that resulted in an objection from CAMRA at the time. However it was eventually deemed as acceptable as there appeared to be no historical reason for the unusual name 'The New Found Out'. In July 1999 the property was bought by Punch Taverns. There were then a number of licensees up to its closure in February 2004. It was then refurbished and reopened in July 2004 as 'The Well', finally closing in March 2010.

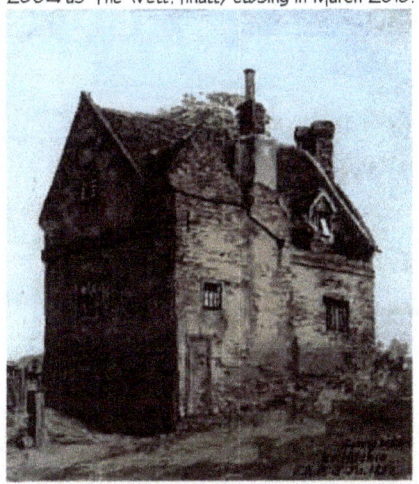

fig. 1   Sunnyside, near Hitchin, 1892, by Evacustes A. Phipson

"The Well", 181 Stevenage Road, Hitchin, Hertfordshire
Design & Access Statement

5. The building has been much altered, particularly during the 20th century. It appears from the above painting (fig. 1) that there was a staircase tower and large chimney stack on the south side of the building, but no trace of these remain. A two storey extension was built on the south side during the early part of the 20th century (see photograph below, fig. 3). Of the original building, most of its south wall has been removed at ground floor, both gables have been rebuilt and dormer windows have been inserted into to the north roof slope. Two gabled single storey extensions were built in 1978 onto the north wall and a third added in the mid 1980s. There is a further two storey extension on the south side of the building which wraps round the west side as single storey, built in 1978, with a large dormer window added in about 1985. A Porch was added to the west elevation in 1978, altered in 2004. Part of the brickwork has been coated with a cream resin/paint material which is unattractive and is unlikely to be able to be removed without causing damage to the brickwork, but fortunately this has not been applied to the brickwork of the original building (although there is a painted rendered plinth on the west elevation).

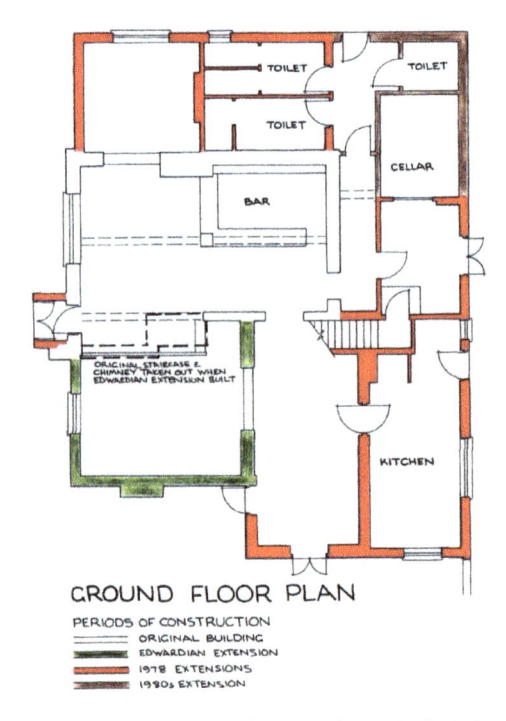

fig. 2 Diagram showing the phases of extension to the building

"The Well", 181 Stevenage Road, Hitchin, Hertfordshire
Design & Access Statement

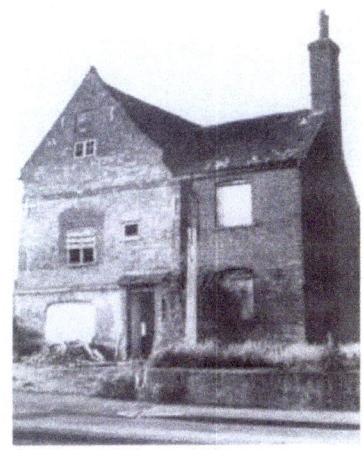

fig. 3 The building circa 1970

6. The planning history is set out in the appendix to this report.

The Proposals

7. It is proposed that the building be converted to residential use by dividing it vertically on the line of the original building to form two houses.

8. The brickwork to the original part of the building is in very poor condition. It is only visible on the west gable (below the gable parapet which has been rebuilt) and to the north elevation above the roofs of the later extensions. It is proposed that it be repaired by removing the cement facings which have been applied and replacing these damaged bricks and other spalled bricks with second-hand bricks to match. Damaged bricks will be turned and reused if their internal faces are useable. The brickwork to be pointed in lime mortar on completion of these repairs. The rendered plinth will be retained.

9. The brickwork to the later extensions will be retained as it is apart from the parts to the west and south elevations which have been coated with a textured resin film. Experience has shown that it is not possible to remove this coating and restore the brickwork so it is proposed that these walls be rendered in a cement/lime mix, wood floated flat and painted with a light cream masonry paint. The end of the parapet to the eastern end of the gable of the single storey to the north elevation to be rebuilt where cracked away from the remainder.

10. The existing Porch on the west elevation is to be removed together with the patch of Fletton brick infill adjoining and a pair of doors inserted with a new brick arch to match the existing arches over.

11. The existing roofs are to be stripped and their plain tiles saved for reuse. Roofs to be re-tiled reusing the existing tiles plus additional second-hand tiles to match as necessary over

"The Well", 181 Stevenage Road, Hitchin, Hertfordshire
Design & Access Statement

"Tyvek" breathing sarking membrane and "Thinsulex" insulating film. Fascias and barge boards to be replaced. The bargeboards on the recent phase of building are very deep and applied directly to the brickwork, giving an unsightly appearance. The detailing of their replacements will be appropriate to the building.

12. The existing windows will be retained and repaired as necessary. Additional windows and doors to be in painted softwood as shown.

13. An informal discussion has taken place with your Conservation Officer and a copy of his Consultation Document dated 15th April is attached. It will be seen that he was happy with the principle of sub-division and the line of the proposed separation.

14. It is proposed that there will be a subsequent application for additional residential development on the site, possibly the construction of a pair of cottages on the redundant car parking area, following further discussion with your Conservation Officer. The restoration and conversion of the existing building is not dependant on the construction of additional development and the applicants wish to obtain consent for these works now so that they can be progressed while additional development is being considered.

15. There will be benefits to the occupants of Alpine Close and the adjoining Cottages on Stevenage Road by the ceasing of the commercial use of the building and the change of use to residential, by way of reduced noise, traffic and disruption.

16. Vehicular and pedestrian access will remain as existing from Alpine Close and the pedestrian gate onto Stevenage Road.

17. The historical research has shown that there is no indication that there has been any use of the site which would give rise to contamination. A copy of the "Passed" certificate from Sitecheck Assess is attached. The site is not in an area of flood risk.

"The Well", 181 Stevenage Road, Hitchin, Hertfordshire
Design & Access Statement

Photographs of the Property (taken March 2010)

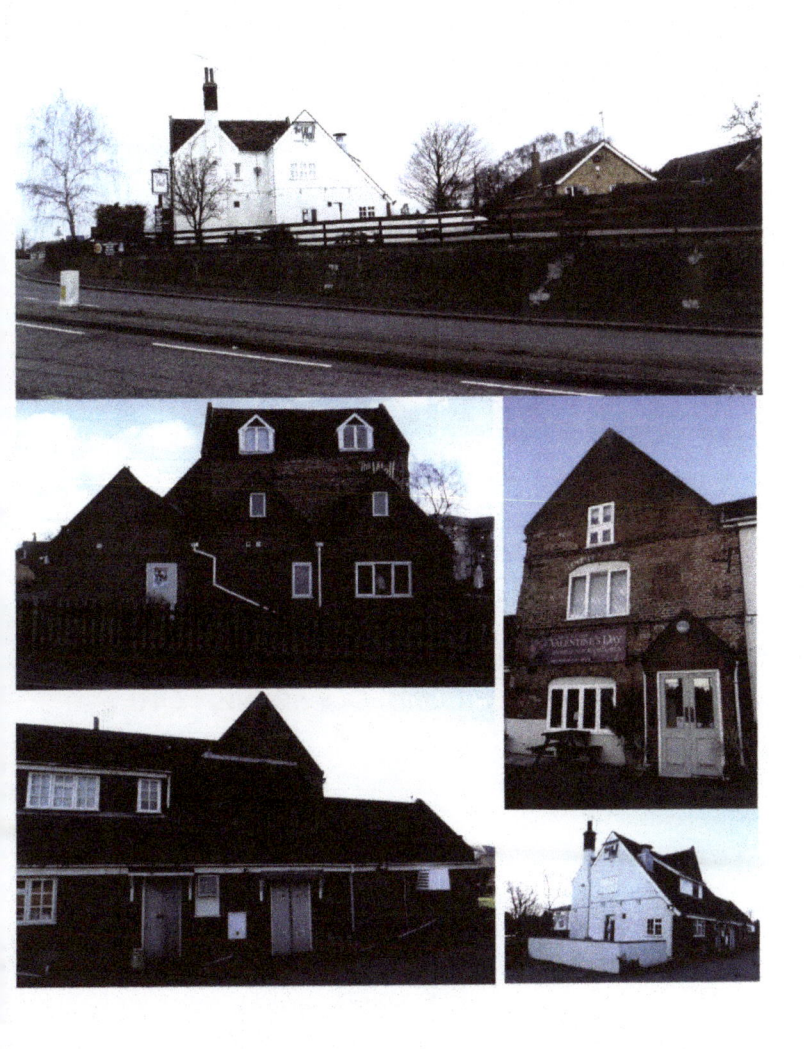

END NOTES

Chapter One

1. Camus,Albert *The Plague.* London. Penguin.1966

2. Buckinghamshire Archives. https://www.buckscc.gov.uk/services/culture-and-leisure/buckinghamshire-archives/online-resources/

3. Acheson,Donald *Public Health in England: the Report of the Committee of Inquiry into the Future Development of the Public Function.* London H.M.S.O. 1988

4. Evelyn,John *Fumifugium.* London. W.Godbid 1661 https://www.google.co.uk/books/edition/Fumifugium/jKY_AQAAMAAJ?hl=en&gbpv=1&printsec=frontcover#spf=1615541079649

5. Banduin,Philip Translated by T.B. & M. Greenhalgh. *Wars and Discoveries.* OREP Editions 2000 p.38

Chapter Two

1. Wilkes, John *History Revealed.* December 2015. Issue.23:p.55

2. Duncan, C.J.; Scott,S. *What caused the Black Death?* British Medical Journal. Postgraduate

Medical Journal Liverpool University. sscottliverpool.ac.uk (https://pmj.bmj.com/content/81/955/315) Accessed 12/03/2021

3. Zeigler, Philip. *The Black Death.* Stroud,Glos. Sutton Publishing. 1969

4. Hatcher, John. *The Black Death.* London. Weidenfeld & Nicholson. 2008 p.57

5. Kiernan, Thomas, Lohoar-Self, Finlay & Jenkinson, Cliff. *Ashwell Church Graffitti.* Ashwell Museum http://www.ashwellmuseum.org.uk/page_id__147.aspx?path=0p4p (accessed 12/03/2021)

6. Porter, Roy. *Blood and Guts: A Short History of Medicine.* London. Penguin. 2002. p.136-7.

7. Stevens-Crawshaw, Jane. *Plague Hospitals.* London. Ashgate Publishing Ltd. 2012 p.12

Chapter Three

1. Wootton, David. *Bad Medicine.* Oxford. Oxford University press. 2006. p.125

2. Ibid. p.119

3. Ibid p.129

4. Sherwood, Thomas. *The Charitable Pestmaster, or The Cure of The Plague.* London. Printed by A.N. for John Francklin. 1641

5. Porter, Stephen. *Disease and the City:*

Seventeenth Century *Plague.* Gresham College, London. 29 October 2001

6. Bradley, Leslie. *The Plague Reconsidered.* Derbyshire. Local population Studies. 1977

7. Ibid

8. Ibid

9. Chalmers, A.K. *Report on certain causes of plague occurring in Glasgow.* Glasgow, Uk. Robert Anderson. 1901.

10. Dean, K. *Royal Society of Open Science.* London. Royal Society Publishing. January 2019

11. Shrewbury, J. F. D. *A History of Bubonic Plague in the British Isles.* Cambridge. Cambridge University press. 1970 p. 448

12. Crawford Adams, John. *Shakespeare's Physic.* London. Royal Society of Medicine. 1989 p. 55

13. Bradley, Leslie. *A Plague Reconsidered.* Derbyshire. Local population Studies. 1977

14. Rideal, Rebecca. *1666 Plague War and Hellfire.* London. John Murray 2016

15. Healy, Margaret. *Discourses of the Plague in Early Modern London.* Epidemic Disease in London Series. Centre for Metropolitan History. 1993 pp.19-34

16. Defoe, Daniel. *Journal of a Plague Year.*

London. Folio Society edition. 1960 p.43

17. Ibid p.145

18. Zeigler, Philip. *The Black Death.* Gloucestershire. Sutton Publishing. 1969.

19. Evans, Jennifer & Read, Sara. *Maladies and Medicine. Exploring health and healing. 1540-1740.* Barnsley, S Yorkshire. Pen and Sword. 2017

20. Ibid

21. Creighton, Charles. *A History of Epidemics in Britain. AD 664 to the Extinction of Plague.* Cambridge. (Forgotten Books.2017) Cambridge University Press. 1891.

22. Defoe, Daniel p.57

23. Ratovonjato J et al. *Yersinia pestis in pulex irritans fleas during plague outbreak in Madagascar* Emerging Infectious Diseases. 20; p.1414-1415

24. (Piarroux R et al. *Plague epidemics and lice. Democratic Republic of Congo.* Emerging Infectious Diseases. 19. p.505-506)

Chapter Four
1. Green, Dr. Matthew. *A travel guide through time.* London. Penguin. 2015 p.180

2. https://archive.org/details/mobot31753000817749/page/ (accessed 10

Jan 2021).

3. https://penelope.uchicago.edu/pseudodoxia/pseudodoxia.shtml *Sir Thomas Browne and the Plague.* Journal of Early Modern Studies. Firenze University Press. Manfred Pfister. July 2020 Sir Thomas Browne. Sir G Keynes. 25 Dec 1965. BMJ. Vol.2. No.5477.pp.1505-1510

4. Steadman, Helen *Widdershins.* London. Impress Books. 2917

5. Cawthorne, Nigel *The Curious Cures of Old England.* London. Portrait Publishing. 2005 p.98

6. Defoe, Daniel. *Journal of a Plague Year.* London. Folio Society edition. 1960 p.180

7. Watson, G. *A Study in Therapeutics.* London. The Wellcome Historical Library. 1966 https://www.ncbi.nlm.nih.gov/pmc/articles/PMC1884566/#__sec5title (accessed 7 April 2021)

8. Evans, Jennifer & Read, Sara. *Maladies and Medicine. Exploring health and healing. 1540-1740.* Barnsley, S Yorkshire. Pen and Sword. 2017

9. Ross, Cathy & Clark, John. *London. The Illustrated History.* London. Penguin. 2008 p.122

10. Eyre, Hermione. *Viper Wine.* London. Jonathan Cape.2014

11. Defoe, D p.27

12. Porter, Stephen. *Disease and the City: Seventeenth Century Plague.* Gresham College, London. 29 October 2001

13. Defoe, D p.68

14. Ibid

15. Ibid p.170

16. Creighton, Charles. *A History of Epidemics in Britain Ad 664 to the extinction of plague.* Cambridge. Cambridge University Press. 2017.

17. Uglow, Jenny. *A Gambling Man. Charles 11 and the Restoration.* London. Faber & Faber. 2009 p.330

18. Leasor, James. *The Plague and the Fire.* London. George Allen & Unwin Ltd. 1962. P.41

19. London School of Hygiene and Tropical Medicine.

Chapter Five
1. Rawcliffe, Carole. *Urban Bodies.* Woodbridge, Suffolk. Boydell Press. 2013.

2. https://en.wikipedia.org/wiki/Lazaretto (accessed 17 March 2021)

3. Rawcliffe, Carole. *Urban Bodies.* Woodbridge. Boydell Press. 2013. p.32

4. Porter, Stephen. *Shakespeare's London.* Stroud, Gloucestershire. Amberley. 2011 p.210

5. Evelyn, John. *The Diary of John Evelyn. 1650-1672 Edn.* E.S. de Beer. Vol.3 Oxford. Oxford University Press. 1955 https://www.oxfordscholarlyeditions.com/view/10.1093/actrade/9780198187509.book.1/actrade-9780198187509-book-1 (accessed 17 March 2021)

Chapter Six

1. Rawcliffe, Carole. *Urban Bodies.* Woodbridge, Suffolk. Boydell Press. 2013. p.129

2. Tannahill, Reay. *Food in History.* London. Penguin Books. 1973

3. Tindall, Gillian. *The Tunnel Through Time.* London. Chatto & Windus. 2016 p. 92-3

4. ibid p.93

5. Champion, Justin. *Epidemic Disease in London.* Centre for Metropolitan History Working Papers Series No.1 1993 p.35-52

6. Ackroyd, Peter. *London the Biography.* London. Vintage Press. 2000 p.556-558

7. Ibid p.557

8. Barton, Nicholas. *The Lost Rivers of London.* London. Phoenix House Ltd. Leicester

University Press. 1962 p.107

9. Leapman, Michael. *London's River.* London. Pavilion Books 1991 p.120

10. Ibid p.107

11. Picard, Liza *Dr. Johnson's London.* London. Phoenix Publishing. 2000 p.10

12. Ibid p.11

13. Wootton, David. *Bad Medicine.* Oxford. Oxford University Press. 2006. P.280

14. Rawcliffe, Carole. *Urban Bodies.* Woodbridge, Suffolk. Boydell Press. 2013. P.353

Chapter Seven

1. Creighton, Charles. *A History of Epidemics in Britain Ad 664 to the extinction of plague.* Cambridge. Cambridge University Press. 2017.

2. Bede's Ecclesiastical History https://www.documentacatholicaomnia.eu/03d/0627-0735,_Beda_Venerabilis,_Ecclesiastical_History_Of_England,_EN.pdf (Accessed 19 March 2021)

3. Creighton, Charles. *A History of Epidemics in Britain Ad 664 to the extinction of plague.* Cambridge. Cambridge University Press. 2017.

4. Clay, Rotha Mary. *Medieval Hospitals of England.* London. Methuen & Co. 1909 http://

www.historyfish.net/clay/mh_chapter_four.pdf

5. Poore, G.V. *London, Ancient and Modern: from the Sanitary and Medical Point of View.* The Project Gutenberg. Cassell & Co. 1889. P.37/128. June 2017 e-book.

6. Creighton, Charles. *A History of Epidemics in Britain Ad 664 to the extinction of plague.* Cambridge. Cambridge University Press. 2017. p.314

7. Cawthorne, Nigel. *The Curious Cures of Old England.* London. Portrait Publishing. 2005. p.96

8. Creighton, Charles. *A History of Epidemics in Britain Ad 664 to the extinction of plague.* Cambridge. Cambridge University Press. 2017. P.322

9. Ibid p.320

10. Simon Kellwaye cited in Creighton, Charles. P.356

11. Ibid p.456

12. Ibid p.466

13. Healy, Margaret. *Discourses of the Plague in Early Modern London.* Epidemic Disease in London Series. Centre for Metropolitan History. 1993 pp.19-34

14. Creighton, Charles p.660

15. Ibid p.647

16. Sloane, M.S. no.349. *An Experimental Relation of the Plague.* William Boghurst. London 1666

17. Walker, Julian. *How to Cure the Plague and Other Curious Remedies.* London. The British Library. 2013. P.132

18. Poore, G.V. *London, Ancient and Modern: from the Sanitary and Medical Point of View.* The Project Gutenberg. Cassell & Co. 1889. P.37/128. June 2017 e-book.

19. Lincoln, Margarette ed. *Samuel Pepys' Plague, Fire, Revolution.* London. Thames & Hudson. p.64

20. Tinniswood, Adrian. *By Permission of Heaven.* London. Jonathan Cape. 2003

21. Tindall, Gillian. *The House by the Thames.* London. Pimlico. 2007 p.51

22. Trease, Geoffrey. *Samuel Pepys and his world.* Book Club Associates. 1972

23. Pierce, Patricia. *Old London Bridge.* Headline Book Publishing. 2001. P.198-203

24. Trease, Geoffrey. p.72

25. Tomalin, Claire. *Samuel Pepys: The Unequalled Self.* London. Penguin Books. 2002. P.170

26. Porter, Stephen. *London's Plague Years.* Stroud, Gloucestershire. Tempus Publishing. 2005

Chapter Eight
1. Clifford, John. *Eyam Plague 1665-1666.* Sheffield. The Print Centre. J.G. Clifford. 1989

2. Clifford, J.G.; Clifford, F. *Eyam Parish Register. 1630-1700.* Chesterfield, Derbyshire. Derbyshire RecordsSociety. 1993 p.9

3. Raoult, D et al. *Plague, History and Contemporary Analysis.* Journal of Infection. 2013 66. P.18-26

4. Whittles, L.K. & Didelot, X. *Epidemiological Analysis of the Eyam Plague Outbreak of 1665-1666.* Proceedings of the Royal Society. 283.20160618. 2016

5. Spitale, Giovanni. *Covid-19 and the Ethics of quarantine: A lesson from the Eyam Plague. University of Zurich.* Medicine, Health Care and Philosophy. 23. December 2020

6. Didelot, Xavier. *Heroic Sacrifice or Tragic Mistake? Revisiting the Eyam Plague, 350 years on.* London. The Royal Statistical Society. Significance. October 2016. p.20-24

7. Ibid

8. Brooks, Geraldine. *Year of Wonders.* London. Fourth Estate. Harper Collins. 2001.

Chapter Nine

1. Leasor, James. *The Plague and the Fire.* London. George Allen and Unwin Ltd. 1962. p.142

2. Ibid p.180

3. Molloy, Joseph Fitzgerald. *Royalty Restored – London under Charles 11* Book on Demand. Vol.1.Ch X1. 2013

4. Leasor, p. 37

5. Clout, Hugh. *History of London.* The Times. Times Books. London. Harper Collins. 2007

6. Leasor p.24

7. Ibid p.26

8. Parker, Geoffrey. *Global Crisis.* London. Yale University Press. New Haven. 2013 p.629

9. Barnett, Richard. *Sick City.* London. Wellcome Trust. 2008 .p.16

10. Johnson, Ben. *The Alchemist.* https://en.wikipedia.org/wiki/The_Alchemist_(play) *(accessed 20 March 2021)*

11. Sick City p.17-18

12. Picard, Liza. *Restoration London.* London. Phoenix. 2003 p.92

13. Ibid p.93

14. The Royal Hospitals NHS Trust. *St. Bartholomew's Hospital. Nine centuries of Healthcare.* 1997 p.37-38

15. Ogg, David. *England in the Reign of Charles 11.* Oxford. Clarendon Press. 1934

16. Porter, Stephen. *Disease and the City. Seventeenth Century Plague.* London. Gresham College. October 2001 https://www.gresham.ac.uk/lecture/transcript/print/17th-century-plague/ (accessed 20 March 2021)

17. Leasor, p.75

18. Ibid

19. Orders Conceived and Published by the Lord Mayor and Aldermen of the City of London concerning the infection of the Plague 1665. https://quod.lib.umich.edu/e/eebo/A53403.0001.001?view=toc (accessed 20 March 2021)

20. Defoe, Daniel. *Journal of a Plague Year.* London. Folio Society edition. 1960 p.30

21. Green, Dr. Matthew. *London. A Travel Guide Through Time.* London. Penguin. 2015 p.169

22. Leasor. P.28

23. Slack, Paul. *The Impact of Plague in Tudor and Stuart England.* London. Clarendon press. Routledge & Paul. 1985.

24. Defoe. P.41

25. Barnett, Richard. *Anatomy of a City.* London. Wellcome Trust. 2008. p.37

26. Evans, Jennifer & Read, Sara. *Maladies and*

*Medicine. Exploring health and healing. 1540-1740.*Barnsley, S Yorkshire. Pen and Sword. 2017

27. Ross, Cathy & Clark, John. *London. The Illustrated History.* London. Penguin. 2008 p.122

28. Defoe, Daniel p.31

29. Black, Winston. *The Plague. All About History.* Bournemouth. Future Publishing Ltd. 12 December 2019. p.28-37

30. Uglow, Jenny. *A Gambling Man. Charles 11 and the Restoration.* London. Faber & Faber. 2009

31. Lincoln, Margaret. Editor. *Plague, Fire, Revolution.* London. National Maritime Museum. Thames & Hudson. p.130

32. Smith, Stephen. *Underground London.* London. Abacus. 2004. p.196-197

33. Latham, R.C & Matthews, W (editors) *The Diary of Samuel Pepys.* Vol. V1 1665 p.181

34. Leasor, James p.30

35. Ibid p.31

36. Defoe, Daniel p.37

37. Leasor, James p.103

38. Defoe, Daniel p.137

39. Leasor, James p.110

40. The National Archives. https://www.nationalarchives.gov.uk/education/resources/great-plague/source-2/ (accessed 20 March 2021)

41. Harding, Vanessa. *Burial of the Plague Dead in Early Modern London.* Epidemic Disease in London edn. Champion, J. Centre for Metropolitan History Working Paper Series. No.1 1993. Pp.53-64

42. Lincoln, Margaret. Editor. *Plague, Fire, Revolution.* London. National Maritime Museum. Thames & Hudson p.133

43. Morant,, Philip. *The History and antiquities of the most ancient town and borough of Colchester, in the County of Essex.*US.Gale Ecco. Print Editions. 2010

44. Martin, G.W. *The Plague in Colchester.* Essex Countryside. Winter 1956/7. P.56

45. Gardiner, Juliet & Wenborn, Neil (editors). *The History Today Companion to British History.* Collins and Brown. 1995 p.352

46. Tinniswood, Adrian. *By Permission of Heaven.* London. Jonathan Cape. 2003

Chapter Ten

1. Chippingdale, S.D. *The Chiltern Hills and Dales in certain of their natural Aspects.* 1910. https://journals.sagepub.com/doi/

abs/10.1177/003591571000300103

2. Ibid

3. Marmoy, C.F.A. *The Pest House: 1681-1717: predecessor of the French Hospital.* London. Proceedings of the Huguenot Society. XXV (4). 1992. p.385-399

4. Poore, George V. *London, Ancient and Modern from the sanitary and medical point of view.* e Book. The Project Gutenberg. Cassell & Co. 2017.

5. Black, Nick. *Walking London's medical History.* London. The Royal Society of Medicine Press. 2006 p.60

6. Marmoy, C.F.A. p.385

7. Arnold, Catherine. *Necropolis. London and its Dead.* London. Pocket Books. 2006

8. Black, Nick p.59

9. Bryant, Arthur. *Samuel Pepys.* Cambridge University Press. The Fontana Library. 1935 p.51

10. Latham, R.C. & Matthews, W. (ed) *The Diary of Samuel Pepys.* Volume V1. 1885. p.162

11. British History Online: (BHO) *Old and New London.* Vol.4. London. Cassell & Galpin. 1878

12. Newman, K.L.S. *Shutt Up, Bubonic Plague and Quarantine in early Modern England.* Journal of Social History. Vol.45. no.3.

2012.p.830 https://www.british-history.ac.uk/survey-london/vols31-2/pt2/pp196-208

13. Arnold, Catherine. Necropolis

14. Thornbury, Walter. *Stepney in Old and new London.* Vol.2.London. 1878.p.137-142 http://www.british-history.ac.uk/old-new-london/vol2/pp.137-142

15. Kennedy, Beverley. *Rickmansworth Historical Review.* Issue 3. June 2014. P.5-10

16. Chippingdale, S.D. https://journals.sagepub.com/doi/pdf/10.1177/003591571000300103 (accessed 24 March 2021)

17. Ibid. https://journals.sagepub.com/doi/pdf/10.1177/003591571000300103 (accessed 24 March 2021)

18. https://www.british-history.ac.uk/vch/herts/vol2/pp323-328

19. Nunn, J.B. *The Book of Watford.* Watford. Publishing Pageprint Ltd. 1987 p.69,101

20. https://www.chipperfield.org.uk/2006/11/02/care-of-the-poor-and-sick-in- chipperfield.html (accessed 24 March 2021)

21. Deddington history online https://www.deddington.org.uk/community/deddington-charity-estates/pest-house-field/ (accessed 24 March 2021)

22. [www.redbournvillage.org.uk/east-common-the-pest-house]

23. Newman, K.L.S. *Shutt Up: Bubonic Plague and Quarantine in Early Modern England.* Journal of Social History. Vol.45. no.3. p.812-830. 2012

24. https://www.british-history.ac.uk/vch/herts/vol2/pp424-432 (accessed 25 March 2021)

25. https://www.british-history.ac.uk/vch/herts/vol2/pp432-438 (accessed 25 March 2021)

26. https://www.british-history.ac.uk/old-new-london/vol6/pp521-528 (accessed 25 March 2021)

27. https://www.british-history.ac.uk/vch/essex/vol5/pp114-127 (accessed 25 March 2021)

28. https://www.eppingforestdc.gov.uk/wp-content/uploads/2019/01/Epping-Historic-Town-Project-ECC-1999.pdf (accessed 25 March 2021)

29. http://faded-london.blogspot.com/2011/02/putney-pest-houses.html (accessed 25 March 2021)

30. Lysons, Daniel. *The Environs of London. Vol.1.* London. County of Surrey. 1792

31. Jones, A.G.E. *The Great Plague in Ipswich.1665- 1666.* P.75-89 1958

32. Ibid

33. https://www.british-history.ac.uk/rchme/herts/pp256-311 (accessed 26 March 2021)

34. https://www.british-history.ac.uk/vch/herts/vol3/pp441-458#h2-0001 (accessed 25 March 2021)

35. https://www.british-history.ac.uk/vch/herts/vol2/pp314-317#h2-0001 (accessed 25 March 2021)

Chapter Eleven

1. Historic England. https://historicengland.org.uk/listing/the-list/list-entry/1268981 (accessed 26 March 2021)

2. Little Hadham Parish News. October 2018. www.littlehadham-pc-gov.uk

3. http://www.workhouses.org.uk/Henley/ (accessed 26 March 2021)

4. Crook, Ruth. *Victims of the Plague were sent to the Pest House.* Grantham Journal. 24 January 2015

5. West Malling – Puckle Cottage. Country Life. 27 October 2014. https://www.countrylife.co.uk/property/country-houses-for-sale-and-property-news/puckle-cottage-kent-64630

6. Gadd, Pat & Pigram, Ron. *Hitchin Inns and Incidents.* Hitchin. 2014. https://www.mattporter.com/wp-content/uploads/2019/11/Hitchin-Inns-and-Incidents.pdf file:///C:/Users/Wall/Downloads/Well%20DAS.pdf (accessed 3 April 2021)

7. Hampshire History. https://www.hampshire-history.com/odiham-pest-house/ (accessed 20 January 2021)

8. Curtis Museum. https://www.hampshireculture.org.uk/sites/default/files/inline-files/PestHouses.pdf (accessed 13 February 2021)

9. https://www.geograph.org.uk/photo/442613 (accessed 26 March 2021)

10. Pest House and Plague in Seventeenth Century in Hungerford. Aspects of the early History of Hungerford. 2009. Norman Hidden}

11. https://www.hungerfordvirtualmuseum.co.uk/index.php/publications (accessed 26 March 2021)

12. Victoria County History. 1990. Vol 12. A History of the County of Oxford

13. Bedfordshire Archives and Records Services. https://bedsarchives.bedford.gov.uk/CommunityHistories/Tebworth/HillCottageTebworth.aspx (accessed 29 March 2021)

14. https://en.wikipedia.org/wiki/Framlingham_Castle (accessed 29 March 2021)

15. https://www.eastmeonhistory.net/pest-house/ (accessed 24 March 2021)

Chapter Twelve
1. Currie, Margaret R. *Fever Hospitals and Fever Nurses.* Oxford. Routledge. p.1
2. McGuiness, Paul (editor) *Timeline The History of Medicine.* History Revealed. Issue 19. August 2015. p.71
3. Currie, Margaret. p.4
4. History Revealed. p.74
5. Parish Nursing Ministries UK. https://parishnursing.org.uk (accessed 31 March 2021)
6. Willett, Jo. *The Pioneering Life of Mary Wortley Montagu.* Barnsley, South Yorkshire. Pen and Sword. 2021
7. Halliday, Stephen. *The Great Filth.* London. Sutton Publishing. 2007 p.5
8. Ayers, G.M. *England's first state hospitals and the metropolitan Asylums Board.* London. Wellcome Institute.
9. Currie, Margaret p.15
10. British Medical Journal (BMJ) *The metropolitan smallpox hospitals. 1886. pp. 361,707 https://www.bmj.com/content/1/1379/1246 (accessed 31 March 2021)*
11. West Watford History Group. www.westwatfordhistorygroup.org
12. Johnson, Steven. *The Ghost* Map. London.

Penguin. 2006. p.123

13. Nunn, J.B. *The Book of Watford.* Watford. Publishing Pageprint Ltd. 1987 p.101

14. Newman, Dr. Vivien & Smyth, Catherine. *Nursing Through Shot and Shell.* London. Pen and Sword. 1988. p.8

15. Currie p.31

16. Ibid p.33

17. Bauduin, Phillipe *Wars and Discoveries.* Gloucester. OREP. 2008. p.43

18. History revealed p.75

19. Currie p.61

20. Picard, Liza. *Elizabeth's London.* London. Phoenix. 2003 p.104

21. Currie p.131

22. McEwen, Yvonne. *In the Company of Nurses: the History of the British Army.* Edinburgh. Edinburgh University Press Ltd. 2014. p.73

23. Currie p.199

24. Whitty, Chris. *Vaccination.* Gresham College Lecture Series. 2021

Chapter Thirteen

1. Hearth Tax. National Archives. https://www.nationalarchives.gov.uk/help-with-your-research/research-guides/taxation-

before-1689/ (accessed 1 April 2021)

2. Office for National Statistics. https://www.ons.gov.uk/peoplepopulationandcommunity/healthandsocialcare/conditionsanddiseases (accessed 1 April 2021)

3. Social Distancing – Covid 19 https://www.nhs.uk/conditions/coronavirus-covid-19/social-distancing/what-you-need-to-do/ (accessed 1 April2021)

4. Chartered Institute of Personnel and Development. CIPD. London. https://www.cipd.co.uk/knowledge/fundamentals/emp-law/employees/furlough#gref (Accessed 1 April 2021)

5. Office for National Statistics. *Ethnic Differences in Coronavirus (COVID – 19) mortality during the first two waves of the pandemic.* London. https://www.ons.gov.uk/news/news/ethnicdifferencesincoronaviruscovid19mortalityduringthefirsttwowavesofthepandemic (accessed 1 April 2021)

6. Hussain, A.N. et al. National Institute for Health NIH. Elsevier Pub. Health Emergency Collection. *Role of testosterone in COVID-19 patients – A double edged sword?* Published online. November 2020. 144.

7. First. Local Government Association (LGA) November 2020. No.653. p.5

8. Ibid

Chapter Fourteen

1. Oldstone, Michael. *Viruses, Plagues and History.* Oxford. Oxford University Press. 1998 p.193

2. Jones, Kate. *Covid-19: are pandemics becoming more common?* UCL East. London. 16 June 2020. https://www.ucl.ac.uk/ucl-east/news/2020/jun/covid-19-are-pandemics-becoming-more-common (accessed 1 April 2021)

3. (https://www.hsj.co.uk/patient-safety/covid-infections-caught-in-hospital-rise-by-a-third-in-one-week/7029211.article (accessed 18 February 2021)

4. Sylvester, Rachel & Thomson, Alice. *Bingham, Kate. The Times.* December 12 2020 p.46-7

5. Litvack, Leon . Creative Commons License file:///C:/Users/Wall/AppData/Local/Microsoft/Windows/INetCache/IE/8JH2C47L/Charles%20Dickens%20wrote%20about%20the%20diphtheria%20crisis%20of%201856%20%E2%80%93%20and%20it%20all%20sounds%20very%20familiar.html (accessed 20 March 2021)

6. McGuiness, Paul (editor*) Timeline The History of Medicine.* History Revealed. Issue 19. August 2015. p.75

7. World Health Organisation (WHO)

Mythbusters. Coronavirus disease. Advice for the public: Mythbusters. https://www.who.int/emergencies/diseases/novel-coronavirus-2019/advice-for-public/myth-busters (accessed 1 April 2021)

8. Piot, Peter. *No Time to lose. Life in pursuit of deadly viruses.* W.W. Norton & Company. 2012. p.175

Milton Keynes UK
Ingram Content Group UK Ltd.
UKHW020620261123
433289UK00010B/29

9 781835 630235